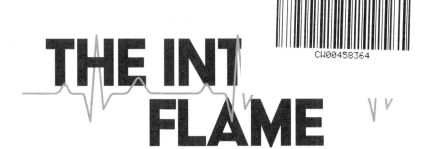

THE INNER FLAME

New insights into silent inflammation, longevity and the science of functional food

BY

DR RODERICK MULGAN

MB, ChB, MPP, LLB (Hons)

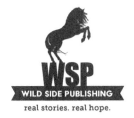

WSP
WILD SIDE PUBLISHING
real stories. real hope.

wildsidepublishing.com

Wild Side Publishing
PO Box 33, Ruawai 0549
Northland, New Zealand
wildsidepublishing.com

Cover design and book layout by Janet Curle, Wild Side Publishing
Proofreading and light copy editing by Sue Beguely, Triplecoil Script

Cataloguing in Publication Data:
Title: The Internal Flame
ISBN: 978-0-473-45573-6 (pbk)
ISBN: 978-0-473-45574-3 (epub)

Subjects: New Zealand Non-Fiction, Medical, Healing, Health.

First printing Benefitz February 2019
International listing 2019 Ingram Spark

DEDICATION

For Sarah, Julia and Emily.

ENDORSEMENTS

Dr Mulgan has written an enticing text in this book. It addresses front-on the health issues faced by a human race living longer than ever before. He then offers explanations and reasons for making diet-based choices that could help us all feel more in control. He has an open and engaging style that also makes you think before you eat.

—Dr Anna Sandiford, BSc(Hons) MSc PhD

An entertaining and informative read—Dr Mulgan has the ability to make complex medical concepts accessible to the general reader. Thought provoking, it has the potential to encourage necessary lifestyle changes. With our population aging there will never be adequate resources to optimally treat all established diseases. Understanding your health and taking preventative and protective measures against the diseases that come with aging has never been more important. I would recommend this book as a resource for all health professionals and any reader with an interest in health and longevity.

—Dr Lawrie Herd MB, ChB MRCGP FRNZCGP DCH

The Internal Flame is an insightful and practical book that anyone wanting longevity and good health for their life should read. It is packed with scientific information that has been diligently researched but written in a way that is engaging and relatable to real life, with advice that can be incorporated into a person's lifestyle with relative ease.

—Karen McMillan, author of *Everyday Strength* and *Unbreakable Spirit*

If you want tips on how to age better, feel healthier, live longer and thrive—then read this book. *The Internal Flame* is an easy-to-read guide on how plants and mindful living can power your health. Certain foods and smart thinking – and living – really can help you to live better. My favourite quote from this book: 'Inheritance is the Hand you are Dealt. Behaviour is How you Play it.'

—Rachel Grunwell, wellness expert and author of *Balance*, columnist for *Good* and *Indulge* magazines

Dr Mulgan has managed to translate years of research and practical medical experience into a well written, easy to understand, and above all—a scientifically based description and solution to one of the greatest issues affecting our health, fitness and longevity. *The Internal Flame* will surely soon become the definitive text for not only health professionals, but more importantly, the general public who will follow his advice and guidelines, improving their general health through the inevitable ageing process. A most compelling read, thought provoking, insightful and inspiring.

—Dr Robert Jones, B.D.S (U. Lond.) L.D.S, R.C.S. Oral, Dental and Cosmetic Surgeon

DR. RODERICK MULGAN

CONTENTS

SECTION 4

ACKNOWLEDGEMENTS

Like most authors (particularly non-fiction ones), I would like to acknowledge that writing is a team sport, and thanks are due to all the people who have played a part. In particular, I greatly appreciate the support and shared vision of Stephen Iorns, my founding partner at LifeGuard Health®.

I am equally grateful for the patience of my wife Sarah, and daughters Julia and Emily, in putting up with my absences, and giving their thoughts on the manuscript as it emerged. The manuscript also benefitted from the attention of my mother Helen, who laboured for hours to find all my grammatical faux pas. I am likewise grateful to Ian Wishart, for expressing his enthusiasm at a crucial time, and for the trouble taken by my editors Matt Turner, Sue Beguely and Victoria Rea.

Thanks also to my publishers Ray and Janet Curle at Wild Side Publishing for unwavering support. The last word of gratitude belongs to LifeGuard® marketing gurus Debra Chantry and Mikael Aldridge for suggesting I write a book in the first place.

FOREWORD

When Roderick Mulgan's manuscript *The Internal Flame* first crossed my desk I felt a huge sense of relief: here was a medical professional singing from the same hymn book I'd found while researching my own health books, *Vitamin D: Is This the Miracle Vitamin?* and *Show Me the Money, Honey: The Truth About Big Pharma's War on Salt, Chocolate, Cholesterol and the Natural Health Products That Could Save Your Life.*

The song is a simple one: our health is linked to our diet and sometimes quite simple food choices can help us reduce our risk of later depending on pharmaceuticals and caregivers to keep us alive.

Humans have lived off the land for aeons and, long before the development of advanced medical science over the past century, our bodies had already developed mechanisms to get the best and avoid the worst of the diets previously available to us. Health researchers are now rediscovering these ancient biological truths. Leaving aside the complex and specific legacy of individual genetics, general good health requires a sensible, balanced and natural diet. Industrialisation has given us packaged, instant, processed foods often made by global conglomerates associated with the very pharmaceutical companies selling the drugs to 'treat' the problems caused by their food products. #Irony.

As consumers we find ourselves bombarded with conflicting messages and studies. 'Go vegan!' shout some, ignoring the fact that a truly vegan diet is unsustainable and unnatural because it is impossible to get all your nutrients from plants in the real pre-industrial world. Veganism depends on processed supplements (industrialisation), or globalised processed farming to provide enough of the obscure plant varieties needed to fill some (but not all) of the nutrient gaps.

Others shout, 'Avoid fat!' or 'Avoid sugar' or 'Avoid carbs', and each of these claims has its own backstory as well.

At the centre of all these issues is inflammation, a body-repair function which works really well for short bursts but is really bad for you if the switch is left on as it is when triggered by diet and environmental stressors. Fortunately, it's within our power to dial inflammation back, once we understand the process.

Books like Dr Mulgan's help ordinary people understand some of the science that will in turn help them make informed health choices for themselves and their families. He has done an exceptional job of clarifying the issues.

No matter which of the various diet 'tribes' you currently adhere to, you will learn something from *The Internal Flame*.

—Ian Wishart, author

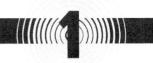

THE WAY OF ALL FLESH

Age, inflammation and functional food

All health-conscious people seek insights that will lead to a long life. So if you want to know what is going to kill you, I can tell you. Perhaps not literally – all rules have exceptions. But if you are in reasonable health and you live in the Western world, you are unlikely to die of infection. Malnutrition, almost certainly not. A car crash is possible, but unlikely. I would wager a large sum you will not be hit by a meteorite. If you fulfil the destiny of most affluent humans in this epoch you will die of your immune system.

I can go further… You may be lucky enough to enjoy good health until the very end of your days, but the odds are against it. As you get older, chances increase that something big – like a stroke, or cancer – will drag down your quality of life. It is not just a question of living to be ninety. It is also a question of being healthy and active as you do it – health span, not just life span.

Well-known healthy options, like eating whole food and exercising, exert a lot of their effect on big diseases by keeping the immune system in balance. Another option in the longevity toolkit, and a major theme of this book, is the developing science of *functional food*.

Which raises the question of what the immune system actually is. You already know its obvious manifestations. If you get a thorn in your

1

finger, it will swell and turn red. It will throb. A bed of pus will form to expel the foreign body, if you haven't pulled it out already. What you are seeing is *inflammation,* the body's defence against outside intruders. Inflammation is the response that repels any threat to your physical integrity by a microorganism such as a bacterium, or a foreign body such as a thorn.

Inflammation also heals the breach afterwards. If you cut yourself, the edges of the wound will turn red as blood vessels swell and proteins are moved in and new cells grow in the gap.

In a nutshell, inflammation is the response of emergency services to a break-in. It is the police, followed by the clean-up crew and the construction teams that repair the damage. It is an elaborate, multifaceted dance of blood cells and specialised proteins. It is as elegant as clockwork, as complex as calculus, as essential as breathing. When it goes right, it saves our lives, and does so many times over in one lifetime. When it goes wrong, it can kill. Usually it does. Most of us will succumb to an inflammation-related disease at the end of our days, and many of us will succumb to one years before that point and live with disability.

That is because inflammation can be activated at the wrong time. It works when it attacks an infectious bacterium. It doesn't work when it smoulders for years, set too low to notice, but quietly burning off blood vessels and healthy organs. That is what happens as we enter our middle years and beyond, and the extent to which it occurs depends on our lifestyle choices.

This book is the story of inflammation and health. It sets out the science behind the big diseases of the latter years. This is mainstream science, well known to doctors and scientists of many disciplines, that underpins what goes wrong as we age, and, in particular, what difference our lifestyle choices make.

But here is the silver lining. Inflammation can be modified. It is almost inevitable you will experience one of these diseases, but what is not inevitable is the timing. How you live and what you eat makes all the difference. Smoking and salmon, walnuts and weight loss, almonds and alcohol, blueberries, white flour, sugar, meditation — each one will turn the thermostat of inflammation up or down.

As do functional foods and their relatives, *nutraceuticals*. This is where the march of anti-inflammatory tactics is leading. Some foods and their derivatives are so effective, almost drug-like, in their capacity to suppress inflammation that seeking them out is indispensable for an optimal strategy. The second half of this book discusses these drug-like options.

Age-related diseases are actually a success story. Two hundred years ago, life expectancy in the First World was around 30 years. That is not to say there were no older people, just that the chance of becoming one was not very good. The large number who died young from infections, childbirth and malnutrition pulled down the average. All that has changed. A century of science, medicine and enlightened public health policies has made all the difference and for the first time in history we live long enough to get old. This means that the diseases associated with getting older are something the average person has to think about. It could be seen as a nice problem to have. Very few people in the past worried about when they might get their first heart attack, nor had any reason to. Today you don't have to expend any energy fending off scurvy or tuberculosis. You have to worry about longevity. And if you worry about longevity, you have to worry about inflammation.

References

Medzhitov, R. (2008). Origin and physiological roles of inflammation. *Nature,* 454.

Riley, J. (2005). Estimates of Regional and Global Life Expectancy, 1800–2001. *Population and Development Review,* 31(3).

2

INFLAMMATION; NUTS AND BOLTS
What inflammation actually is

Even the simplest creatures need some mechanism for defence and repair to stay alive. The earliest shellfish, for instance, threw enzymes and toxins at intruders who breached their shells and patched up the damage afterwards. Something similar can be found in every animal that nature has come up with. Humans and fruit flies share the same genes for it. Inflammation touches everything.

Scholars first noticed inflammation in classical times (the word comes from the Latin for flame). Hippocrates, in the fifth century BC, recognised that it was part of healing. Celsus, a Roman writer who lived between 30 BC and 45 AD, described the four cardinal signs as redness, warmth, swelling and pain. Another Greek writer, Galen, added loss of function. Modern doctors define it the same way.

After the microscope came along in the sixteenth century, scientists got a better look at what was going on. They saw white blood cells that had passed through the walls of blood vessels to the tissue on the other side. They saw new blood vessels growing in healing wounds. In the nineteenth century a German called Rudolph Virchow, the father of modern pathology, described inflammatory cells in cancer and in atherosclerosis, the fat deposits that cause heart attacks. He was ahead of his time. Despite Virchow's towering reputation, the possibility that inflammation may cause cancer and heart attacks lay dormant in medical minds for a hundred and fifty years.

These days the association is widely known and it is the subject of this book. I will attempt to elucidate the connection and, in simple terms, describe how inflammation actually works. Unfortunately, the chemistry is of Olympian complexity and modern research is still chasing many of the details. If you want a challenging read there are thousands of publications available with this sort of thing:[1]

> In healthy individuals, RNA-IC induced interferon (IFN)-α, tumor necrosis factor (TNF)-α, IL-6, IL-8, IFN-γ, macrophage inflammatory protein (MIP)1-α, and MIP1-β production in pDC and NK cell cocultures. IFN-α production was selective for pDCs, whereas both pDCs and NK cells produced TNF-α. IRAK4i reduced the pDC and NK cell-derived cytokine production by 74-95%.

So now you know. Fortunately, the basic process and the main actors can be stated more easily. The inflammatory response runs off specialised proteins such as antibodies and white blood cells which go round and round in your bloodstream waiting for something to happen, like police cars on patrol. They swing into action when local tissues detect a noxious stimulus like a thorn or bacteria, or even just trauma like a sprained ankle. When that happens signalling cells fire proteins towards nearby capillaries. Capillaries are hair-like blood vessels made of flat cells rolled up in tubes with waterproof joins. The signalling molecules tell them to leak, so the joins break down and blood products squeeze through. This is where the swelling, the redness and the heat come from — all the extra volume squeezed out of the blood vessels.

---

1 Hjorton, K., Hagberg, N., Israelsson, E., Jinton, L., Berggren, O., Sandling, J.K., Thörn, K., Mo, J., The DISSECT consortium, Eloranta, M-L., & Rönnblom, L. (2018). Cytokine production by activated plasmacytoid dendritic cells and natural killer cells is suppressed by an IRAK4 inhibitor. *Arthritis Research & Therapy*, 20,238.

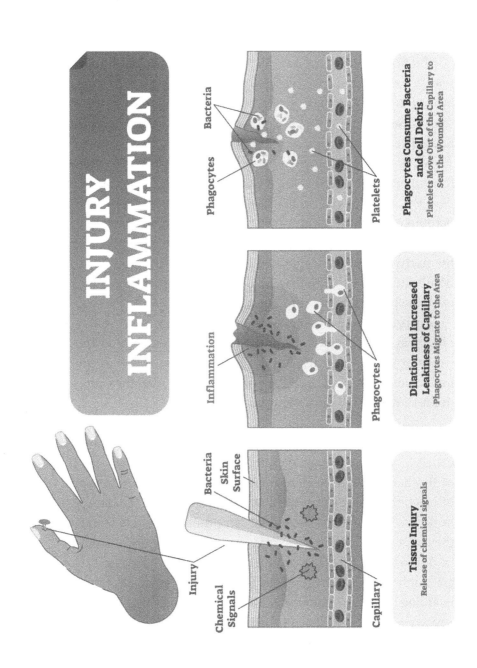

INJURY

INFLAMMATION

Injury

Bacteria
Skin
Surface

Chemical
Signals

Capillary

Tissue Injury
Release of chemical signals

Inflammation

Phagocytes

**Dilation and Increased
Leakiness of Capillary**
Phagocytes Migrate to the Area

Bacteria

Phagocytes

Platelets

**Phagocytes Consume Bacteria
and Cell Debris**
Platelets Move Out of the Capillary to
Seal the Wounded Area

7

The first white blood cells that squeeze themselves into the scene release toxic granules to kill the invader. In fact, the toxic granules kill everything in the area. Collateral damage is all part of it. It is worth it to us to sacrifice some of our tissue, which we can repair, in order to neutralise a threat.

When the shooting has stopped, different white cells swallow the foreign material to neutralise it and carry it away. The process is called *phagocytosis*. The cell wraps itself around the foreign body like an octopus and contains it in a bubble of its own membrane.

Then repair starts (think of a healing cut). Proteins assemble themselves, new cells appear and blood vessels grow through the bomb site to conduct the materials in. (Healing tissue is pink because of all the blood flowing through it).

The process requires immense coordination, which means a system of signals. Every battle group needs its messengers be they radio waves or carrier pigeons, and the inflammatory army has specialised molecules, which are useful to dwell on, because they are a major point of assault for anti-inflammatory therapies. The principal ones are *cytokines*, small proteins that cells use to talk to each other. The cell wanting to send a message – such as 'come and join the fight!' – expels a cytokine which floats off and looks for a receptor on the wall of another cell. It fits itself inside, like a key in a lock, and sets off a train of reactions inside the second cell that tells it what to do. Cytokines don't live long, which is fortunate since things would become messy if they kept on delivering messages long after they were posted.

Some of the messages are carried by *reactive oxygen species*, which are highly unstable, oxygen-based molecules, and which also play a role in killing intruders. They are the same as the ones that cause oxidative stress, a major cause of age-related inflammation, as described further on in The inflammage. You see what I mean about complexity!

In fact, the whole gamut of signals is inflammation's weak point. The functional foods described in the third section of this book often work by knocking out cytokines or oxygen species. There is nothing modern about jamming the enemy's radios.

One characteristic of inflammation that is vital for our story is that it is blunt. Numerous different threats and injuries all provoke the same response: a wave of cells and toxins which kill civilians and soldiers alike, followed by containment and clean-up. It is not a finely tuned attack that pinpoints the threat and escorts it off the premises. It is a grenade, which takes out the invader and everything around it. Soft treatment of an intruder can be fatal, so nature has made the response decisive, with collateral damage as the price to be paid. This is an important consideration when inflammation goes wrong. An outbreak here and there is containable, but when outbreaks multiply in number, which they do as you get older (again, see The inflammage), the repair crews have trouble keeping up. This, in other words, is disease.

References

Granger, D.N., & Senchenkova, E. (2010). Inflammation and the Microcirculation. *San Rafael (CA): Morgan and Claypool Life Sciences,* 2.

Hjorton, K., Hagberg, N., Israelsson, E., Jinton, L., Berggren, O., Sandling, J.K., Thörn, K., Mo, J., The DISSECT consortium, Eloranta, M-L., & Rönnblom, L. (2018). Cytokine production by activated plasmacytoid dendritic cells and natural killer cells is suppressed by an IRAK4 inhibitor. *Arthritis Research & Therapy,* 20,238.

Lushchak, V. (2014). Free radicals, reactive oxygen species, oxidative stress and its classification. *Chemico-Biological Interactions,* 224, 164-175.

McCord, J. (2000). The evolution of free radicals and oxidative stress. *The American Journal of Medicine,* 108(8), 652-659.

Medzhitov, R. (2008). Origin and physiological roles of inflammation. *Nature,* 454(7203), 428-435.

Rubin, E.R., & Reisner, H.M. *In Essentials of Rubin's Pathology* (6th ed). Walter Klewers.

Stix, G. (2007). A malignant flame. *Scientific American.*

Suman, S., Sharma, P., Rai, G., Mishra, S., Arora, D., Gupta, P., & Shukla, Y. (2016). Current perspectives of molecular pathways involved in chronic inflammation-mediated breast cancer. *Biochemical and Biophysical Research Communications,* 472(3), 401-409.

Tousoulis, D., Psarros, C., Demosthenous, M., Patel, R., Antoniades, C., & Stefanadis, C. (2014). Innate and Adaptive Inflammation as a Therapeutic Target in Vascular Disease. *Journal of the American College of Cardiology*, 63(23), 2491-2502.

Ventura, H.O. (2000). Rudolph Virchow and Cellular Pathology. *Clinical Cardiology*, 23, 550-552.

Wilson, C., Finch, C., & Cohen, H. (2002). Cytokines and Cognition—The Case for A Head-to-Toe Inflammatory Paradigm. *Journal of American Geriatrics Society*, 50(12).

˙ Emerging Microbes & Infections (2013); Published online 18 September 2013.

3

THE INFLAMMAGE
The dark side of immunity and age

It is tricky working out why we age. Wear and tear is obviously part of it, but organs can repair themselves, so why can't they keep going? Theorists love getting stuck into this. Why don't we die once we have raised our children, and nature has no further use for us? Is ageing programmed, written into our genes? Is it the way we live, accumulating health or harm from food, toxins and radiation? If so, how far out can frailty be pushed if we do everything right?

Over 300 theories purport to explain ageing. Some of them are wonderfully exotic (tunnelling nanotube supercellularity, for instance), but mainstream thinking comes down to several key themes, one of which is so influential it has its own word: inflammaging. The term was coined at the turn of the century to refer to the way that inflammation goes hand in hand with the business of getting older, and it has captured the imagination of numerous researchers. If everything big and terrible about ageing has the same basis (which looks increasingly likely), then treatments which could knock over multiple diseases in one swoop are on the horizon. Even if a new drug is not close, the inflammage insight can guide lifestyle choices, and fine-tune our efforts to eat and live proactively.

Staying alive in a hostile environment calls for aggressive defences, so nature has equipped us with them. Everyone alive today had ancestors whose immune systems fought off infection and injury until they could raise their children. That was all good when life expectancy was 30 but in the last two centuries medicine, nutrition and town planning – dry houses, treated sewerage – have become so good that most people will get old. That means their immune systems will run much longer than they were designed to. Unfortunately, over-extended immune systems are trouble.

Older people in normal health usually have higher blood levels of the molecules doctors use to measure inflammation. In other words, these molecules or markers are no longer pointing to an illness; they are normal for older cohorts. They can even be used to make predictions. Healthy older people with raised makers lose their health sooner than age-matched people with normal ones.

The issue is largely one of time… As years go by, you accumulate things. Most people could cite memories, books and children, for example. Others could add wine, cars and sports trophies. Your immune system is the same, except that it accumulates insults arising from all the infections and foreign bodies it has grappled with, and the damaged cells it has cleared away. It can cope up to the point when humans used to die; beyond that, it is processing a cumulative stimulus it was not designed for.

Age also visits new stresses such as long-term, low-grade viruses which even healthy people walk around with, and molecules from the gut which becomes leaky over the years (see <u>Bioavailability; Getting past the border guards</u>).

A core concept is oxidative stress which starts with the normal process of turning food into energy. Energy for your body is released when the food you eat meets the oxygen you inhale inside tiny furnaces called *mitochondria*.[1] The reaction is a fire – fuel plus oxygen, like burning a log – and it powers muscle movement, body heat, heart beat and every other thing your body does. Like any other fire, it causes pollution. The pollution from burning food is oxygen free radicals. An oxygen free radical is an unstable molecule based on oxygen, and burning food makes a lot of them.[2] Oxygen atoms are essential to the process, but they get spun out afterwards as waste. Up to three per cent of the oxygen you inhale goes up the mitochondrial chimney as a free radical, and free radicals are trouble. In terms of chemistry, free radicals have unpaired electrons which makes them unstable. They want to rip electrons off other molecules which effectively makes them roving bands of teenage misfits looking to start something. Usually, they start it with other, more sober and sedate molecules like proteins and fats and, most worryingly, DNA. Cells may die if their proteins and fats (fats are cell walls) are roughed up by free radicals, and roughed up DNA can cause cancer.

It is strange to tell, but the breath of life is one of nature's most dangerous molecules. We die in minutes without it but, as with rusty iron and rancid milk, oxygen is the natural world's agent of decay. We would decay too if we could not contain it, so our cells have enzymes that disable free radicals as they appear off the production line. These enzymes stop us rotting as we go about our lives but they struggle on their own. That is the cue for dietary *antioxidants*. Antioxidants

---

1 It all comes down to swapping electrons around. Electrons orbit atoms, and molecules – which are aggregations of atoms – are held together with shared electron orbits. Plants use energy from the sun to drive electrons 'uphill' against their tendency so molecules of water and atmospheric carbon dioxide can be broken up and their atoms rearranged to form long carbon chains (which is what plants are made of), and oxygen gas. When we eat plants, or burn them in the fireplace, or in an engine (petrol is rotten trees), oxygen in the air takes the electrons back and frees the energy.

2 Some terminology: A free radical is a molecule with one or more unpaired electrons in its outer orbit. An oxygen free radical is one based on the oxygen atom. While the oxygen versions are the main free radicals produced by mitochondria, there are also free radicals based on other elements like nitrogen and sulphur. Collectively these molecules, along with other highly unstable ones, are called reactive species.

also disable free radicals. They probably work by boosting our own enzymes, not by attacking free radicals directly – the chemistry is complicated and still being worked out – but undoubtedly they are good for us. Fruits and vegetables are full of antioxidants, and one of the reasons they are the heart, so to speak, of healthy eating. Staying well means cleaning up the pollution.

Free radicals are unavoidable, even in good health, since mitochondrial furnaces are the life force and they have not found any other way of doing it. But your environment makes it worse: UV light on your skin will make free radicals, as will fine particles from vehicle exhausts – which can penetrate your body all the way into mitochondria – and numerous other influences. Cigarettes, radiation, alcohol, junk food and couch potato habits all add to the free-radical burden.

Oxidative stress occurs when free radicals outweigh the forces arrayed against them. Diets deficient in antioxidants will cause it, as will the wrong lifestyle choices. Scientists have compelling data that links oxidative stress with cancer, brain disease, heart pathology and basically all the inflammatory conditions. This is a problem as you get older: your cells produce far more free radicals in old age than in your youth. This is partly because your mitochondria start to malfunction and put out more pollution, like old cars. It is also because the antioxidant forces start to sag.

The picture is not clear cut (it never is) because free radicals have some useful functions as well, and their specific contribution to ageing is debated. Perhaps some tend to help, others tend to harm. It was once widely accepted they were the prime cause of age-related decline but that theory has taken some knocks. Their association with major inflammatory diseases like cancer, rather than ageing per se, is better established.

When macromolecules like fat and DNA are damaged by a free radical rampage they are no longer normal. The immune system thinks they are intruders, and sends in the forces of inflammation to remove them.

Free radicals also turn on the receptors that activate a protein called Nuclear Factor Kappa B (NFκB), which is a master regulator of inflammatory genes and a major point at which inflammation gets stirred up by age. NF-κB manages the reading of around 400 genes that code for cytokines, adhesion molecules, enzymes and all manner of key inflammatory constituents. It is sometimes likened to a smoke alarm: it sits in every cell of your body and when it detects stress or a noxious substance, it elbows its way into the cell's nucleus – the HQ where the DNA lives – and starts shouting orders at the genes of inflammation. When free radicals peter out, the effect on NF-κB is short-lived; when they keep coming, the stimulation becomes permanent.

Furthermore, getting older exposes the system to more and more cells that have reached their natural lifespan. Until the 1960s, experts believed cells were immortal, that you could stick them in a warm bath and they would divide for as long as you fed them. That view was turned upside down in 1961 by a researcher called Leonard Hayflick. He discovered cells will only divide around 60 times (give or take) before they grind to a halt. He had discovered *senescence* or the state of naturally arrested cell division.

Senescence happens largely because *telomeres*, the ends of DNA molecules, get frayed as DNA replicates, which it does every time a cell divides. At some point, these tips become unfit for purpose. There are so many divisions, then that is it. The cell can't divide any more. There is tantalising evidence that telomere length can be preserved by healthy eating. In other words, the length of your telomeres does not follow your age in years; you can hang onto them by doing the right things.

A senescent cell fires off a barrage of inflammatory cytokines to let the system know it needs to be cleared away and the site of its demise repaired. That works well when there are only a few. It is overwhelming when the numbers get too large which, given senescence is a function of time, they are bound to do. When multiplied numerous times, a request for a local clean-up becomes a system-wide overreaction.

Inflammation is made worse by sloppy housekeeping. Cells have mechanisms to sweep away discarded proteins but they become sluggish with age, so the rubbish piles up outside the door and the response it provokes is that much bigger.

Unfortunately, there are consequences when inflammation gets out of hand, and those consequences are the subject of the next few chapters. The inflammage is far from benign, and staying healthy into middle age and beyond has a lot to do with keeping a lid on it. Known healthy tactics such as taking exercise and eating vegetables exert positive effects on the inflammatory balance. This is largely why they are effective, but a question of great interest is whether there is anything else. The hunt is on for a drug that blocks the inflammage, with unthinkable profits for the company that finds one. A parallel and less glamorous enquiry concerns existing natural options. There is respectable evidence that targeting anti-inflammatory fractions of food, and related compounds like spices, could amount to a whole new toolkit in the task of staying well while getting older.

References

Abdali, D., Samson, S.E., & Grover, A.K. (2015). How effective are antioxidant supplements in obesity and diabetes? *Medical Principles and Practice,* 24(3), 201-15.

Ahn, K. S. and Aggarwal, B. B. (2005). Transcription Factor NF-κB: A Sensor for Smoke and Stress Signals. *Annals of the New York Academy of Sciences,* 1056, 218–233.

Alov, P., Tsakovska, I., & Pajeva, I. (2015). Computational Studies of Free Radical-Scavenging Properties of Phenolic Compounds. *Current Topics in Medicinal Chemistry,* 15(2), 85-104.

Baylis, D., Bartlett, D., Patel, H., & Roberts, H. (2013). Understanding how we age: insights into inflammaging. *Longevity & Healthspan,* 2, 8-8.

Berg, D., Youdim, M., & Riederer, P. (2004). Redox imbalance. *Cell and Tissue Research,* 318(1), 201-213.

Birch-Machin, M., & Bowman, A. (2016). Oxidative stress and ageing. *British Journal of Dermatology,* 175, 26-29.

Calcada, D., Vianello, D., & Giampieri, E. (2014). The role of low-grade inflammation and metabolic flexibility in aging and nutritional modulation thereof: a systems biology approach. *Mechanisms of Ageing and Development,* 138-147.

Campisi, J. (2013). Aging, Cellular Senescence, and Cancer. *Annual Review of Physiology,* 75, 685-705.

Candore, G., Caruso, C., & Colonna-Romano, G. (2010). Inflammation, genetic background and longevity. *Biogerontology,* 11(5), 565-573.

Cannizzo, E., Clement, C., Sahu, R., Follo, C., & Santambrogio, L. (2011). Oxidative stress, inflamm-aging and immunosenescence. *Journal of Proteomics,* 74(11), 2313-2323.

Castellani, G.C., Menichetti, G., Garagnani, P., Bacalini, M.G., Pirazzini, C., Franceschi, C., Collino, S., Sala, C., Remondini, D., Giampieri, E., Mosca, E., Bersanelli, M., Vitali, S., do Valle, I.F., Pietro, L., & Milanesi, L. (2016). Systems medicine of inflammaging. *Briefings in Bioinformatics,* 17(3), 527-540.

Chung, H., Cesari, M., Anton, S., Marzetti, E., Giovannini, S., Seo, A., Carter, C., Yu, B., & Leeuwenburgh, C. (2009). Molecular inflammation: Underpinnings of aging and age-related diseases. *Ageing Research Reviews,* 8(1), 18-30.

Coates, P. (2013). In Brief: cell senescence. *The Journal of Pathology,* 230(3), 239-240.

Bertram, C., & Hass, R. (2008). Cellular responses to reactive oxygen species-induced DNA damage and aging. *Biological Chemistry,* 389(3).

Cortese-Krott, M.M., Koning, A., Kuhnle, G.G.C., et al. (2017). The Reactive Species Interactome: Evolutionary Emergence, Biological Significance, and Opportunities for Redox Metabolomics and Personalized Medicine. *Antioxidants & Redox Signaling,* 27(10), 684-712.

Davies, K. (2000). An Overview of Oxidative Stress. *IUBMB Life,* 50(4-5), 241-244.

De Gara, L., Locato, V., Dipierro, S., & de Pinto, M. (2010). Redox homeostasis in plants. The challenge of living with endogenous oxygen production. *Respiratory Physiology & Neurobiology,* 173, S13-S19.

Ershler, W. B. (2007). A gripping reality: oxidative stress, inflammation, and the pathway to frailty. *Journal of Applied Physiology,* 103(1).

Fang, Y., Yang, S., & Wu, G. (2002). Free radicals, antioxidants, and nutrition. *Nutrition*, 18(10), 872-879.

Fogarasi, E., Croitoru, M., Fülöp, I., & Muntean, D. (2016). Is the Oxidative Stress Really a Disease? *Acta Medica Marisiensis*, 62(1).

Forman, H.J., Davies, K.J., & Ursini, F. (2014). How do nutritional antioxidants really work: nucleophilic tone and para-hormesis versus free radical scavenging in vivo. *Free Radical Biology and Medicine*, 66, 24-35.

Franceschi, C., & Campisi, J. (2014). Chronic Inflammation (Inflammaging) and Its Potential Contribution to Age-Associated Diseases. *The Journals of Gerontology Series A: Biomedical Sciences and Medical Sciences*, 69(Suppl_1), S4-S9.

Frasca, D., & Blomberg, B. (2016). Inflammaging decreases adaptive and innate immune responses in mice and humans. *Biogerontology*, 17(1), 7-19.

Freitas-Simoes, T.M., Ros, E., & Sala-Vila, A. (2016) Nutrients, foods, dietary patterns and telomere length: Update of epidemiological studies and randomized trials. *Metabolism*, 65(4), 406-415.

Fulle, S., Protasi, F., Di Tano, G., Pietrangelo, T., Beltramin, A., Boncompagni, S., Vecchiet, L., & Giorgio, F. (2004). The contribution of reactive oxygen species to sarcopenia and muscle ageing. *Experimental Gerontology*, 39(1), 17-24.

Garber, K. (2012). Biochemistry: A radical treatment. *Nature*, 489(7417), S4-S6.

Gonzalez-Freire, M., de Cabo, R., Bernier, M., Sollott, S., Fabbri, E., Navas, P., & Ferrucci, L. (2015). Reconsidering the Role of Mitochondria in Aging. *The Journals of Gerontology Series A: Biomedical Sciences and Medical Sciences*, 70(11), 1334-1342.

Hartley, A-V., Martin, M., & Lu, T. (2017). Aging: Cancer – an unlikely couple. *Aging (Albany NY)*. 9(9), 1949-1950.

Kirkwood, T., & Kowald, A. (2012). The free-radical theory of ageing – older, wiser and still alive. *BioEssays*, 34(8), 692-700.

Larbi, A., Franceschi, C., Mazzatti, D., Solana, R., Wikby, A., & Pawelec, G. (2008). Aging of the Immune System as a Prognostic Factor for Human Longevity. *Physiology*, 23(2),

Lee, J., Koo, N., & Min, D. (2004). Reactive Oxygen Species, Aging, and Antioxidative Nutraceuticals. *Comprehensive Reviews in Food Science and Food Safety*, 3(1).

Liu, Y., Long, J., & Liu, J. (2014). Mitochondrial free radical theory of aging: Who moved my premise? *Geriatrics & Gerontology International*, 14(4), 740-749.

Lushchak, V. (2014). Free radicals, reactive oxygen species, oxidative stress and its classification. *Chemico-Biological Interactions*, 224, 164-175.

McCord, J. (2000). The evolution of free radicals and oxidative stress. *The American Journal of Medicine*, 108(8), 652-659.

Muñoz, A., & Costa, M. (2013). Nutritionally Mediated Oxidative Stress and Inflammation. *Oxidative Medicine and Cellular Longevity*.

Muriach, M., Flores-Bellver, M., Romero, F., & Barcia, J. (2014). Diabetes and the Brain: Oxidative Stress, Inflammation, and Autophagy. *Oxidative Medicine and Cellular Longevity*.

Passaglia, A., Schuch, N., Cestari, M.N., Schuch, J., Frederico, C., Menck, M., Carrião, C., & Garcia, M. (2017). Sunlight damage to cellular DNA: Focus on oxidatively generated lesions. *Free Radical Biology and Medicine,* 107, 110-124.

Petersen, K., & Smith, C. (2016). Ageing-Associated Oxidative Stress and Inflammation Are Alleviated by Products from Grapes. *Oxidative Medicine and Cellular Longevity.*

Poljsak, B., Šuput, D. &, Milisav, I. (2013). Review Article Achieving the Balance between ROS and Antioxidants: When to Use the Synthetic Antioxidants. *Oxidative Medicine and Cellular Longevity.*

Pryor, W., Houk, K., Foote, C., Fukuto, J., Ignarro, L., Squadrito, G., & Davies, K. (2006). Free radical biology and medicine: it's a gas, man!. *AJP - Regulatory, Integrative and Comparative Physiology,* 291(3).

Rafie, N., Golpour Hamedani, S., Barak, F., Safavi, S.M., & Miraghajani, M. (2016). Dietary patterns, food groups and telomere length: a systematic review of current studies. *The European Journal of Clinical Nutrition.*

Rustom, A. (2016). The missing link: does tunnelling nanotube-based supercellularity provide a new understanding of chronic and lifestyle diseases? *Open Biology,* 6(6).

Seals, D., Justice, J., & LaRocca, T. (2016). Physiological geroscience: targeting function to increase healthspan and achieve optimal longevity. *The Journal of Physiology,* 594(8), 2001-2024.

Speakman, J., & Selman, C. (2011). The free-radical damage theory: Accumulating evidence against a simple link of oxidative stress to ageing and lifespan. *BioEssays,* 33(4), 255-259.

Sosa, V., Teresa, M., Somoza, R., Paciucci, R., Kondoh, H., & LLeonart, M. (2013). Oxidative stress and cancer: An overview. *Ageing Research Reviews,* 12(1), 376-390.

Soysal, P., Stubbs, B. et al. (2016), Inflammation and frailty in the elderly: A systematic review and meta-analysis. *Ageing Research Reviews,* 31.

Turkan, I. (2017). Emerging roles for ROS and RNS – versatile molecules in plants. *Journal of Experimental Botany,* 68(16), 4413–4416.

van Deursen, J. (2014). The role of senescent cells in ageing. *Nature,* 509(7501), 439-446.

Viña, J., Borrás, C., & Miquel, J. (2007). Theories of ageing. *IUBMB Life,* 59(4-5), 249-254.

Zhang, J., Rane, G., Dai, X., Shanmugam, M., Arfuso, F., Samy, R., Lai, M., Kappei, D., Kumar, A., & Sethi, G. (2016). Ageing and the telomere connection: An intimate relationship with inflammation. *Ageing Research Reviews,* 25, 55-69.

4

DEALING WITH DESTINY

*The science of changing the future, from the town
that won our hearts*

So if age means inflammation and, as you will read in a few pages, inflammation underpins life's big diseases, the question is whether anything can be done. Can life's health trajectory be changed? You would expect modern medicine to say yes, but it was not always so.

If you leave the city limits of Boston on the east coast of the States, it will take you less than an hour to get to the town of Framingham. There is nothing about Framingham that strikes the eye; it is a one-time factory settlement surrounded by farms with a population of 70,000. It does not figure in popular culture and no high-end tourist attractions make their home there. Yet the modest exterior is misleading, and its legacy to humanity goes unsung. You have experienced its influence even if you have not heard its name, and millions live longer because of the milestone in medical history that is planted there.

In the developed world, most people die of their blood vessels, which means heart attacks and strokes. Anything that keeps critical arteries open would save countless lives, yet for decades many people, including doctors, thought that early death from heart disease was just a lottery. The possibility of intervening did not enter their heads. It is due to Framingham, or more properly, the Framingham Heart Study, that the modern world knows differently.

It took a long time. Doctors have known since the nineteenth century that some aspects of their craft could be studied as patterns. In 1854, for instance, before germs were known to cause disease (meaning before there was an explanation), authorities removed the handle of the water pump in Broad Street, London, because a map of cholera distribution centred on it.[1] A whole branch of medicine, called epidemiology, followed. It was founded on the idea that if disease could arise from the environment then maps and questionnaires and public health records could plumb medical truths as well as microscopes and test tubes. By the 1940s, medical minds started to wonder if non-infectious diseases could be unpicked in the same way. The government, and the insurance industry (which turned its profit on predicting mortality), collected causation details from death certificates and they discovered that the incidence of heart disease was going up. It would be nice to know why.

If age alone brought heart disease on, as many thought, the incidence would be static. Perhaps there were other causes? Perhaps if some people were studied for long enough they could be spotted? It was a novel concept, and a lot of doctors needed convincing. The idea of risk factors and statistical methods beyond infectious diseases was uncharted territory.

A risk factor is simply something that pushes the odds in a certain direction. For example, driving a car with bald tyres is riskier than driving one with proper tread. It does not confer certainty – not every vehicle with bald tyres will crash, and not every smoker will get cancer – so working out what is risky means watching large groups of people for a long time and running their data through complex formulas.

---

1   This episode is often cited as the first recorded example of the precautionary principle, which is the proposition that preventative action against a serious threat should not wait until evidence becomes certain. The principle continues to inform major debates, such as the best response to climate change and genetic modification.

As early as the 1920s the insurance industry, which had money riding on it, knew high blood pressure caused heart disease at levels the medical profession said were normal. Risk resonated with the business world long before it made sense to doctors.

Nevertheless, enquiring minds were intrigued. Franklin Roosevelt, America's wartime president, gave the issue a jolt by dying of a brain bleed while in office. He had suffered for years with high blood pressure and poorly controlled heart failure and at his last summit with Churchill and Stalin, where they mapped out the post-war world, he appeared too ill to hold the line about Eastern Europe. Did blood vessel disease give us the communist bloc? The National Heart Act, passed by Congress in 1948, was in some measure a response to the president's death. The preamble read:

> Whereas the Congress hereby finds and declares that the Nation's health is seriously threatened by diseases of the heart and circulation... it is therefore the policy of the United States to provide for research and control relating to diseases of the heart and circulation in a supreme endeavour to develop speedily more effective means of prevention, diagnosis, and treatment of such diseases.

Wheels started to turn in the Public Health Service 'to study the expression of coronary artery disease in a "normal" or unselected population and to determine the factors predisposing to the development of the disease through clinical and laboratory exam and long term follow-up ...'[2] Framingham, peopled mainly with European blue-collar workers, was judged to be an ideal microcosm of American society and conveniently close to the cardiologists at Harvard.

---

2   Prescient words from the original proposal, written in 1947 by a young officer and physician called Gilcin Meadors. See Mahmood, S.S., Levy, D., et al. (2014). The Framingham Heart Study and the Epidemiology of Cardiovascular Diseases: A Historical Perspective. *Lancet*, 383(9921): 999–1008.

The first subject was enrolled in 1948. (This was quite a good year for health: the World Health Organisation and Britain's National Health Service were born in that year too). Over the next four years the study grew to include 5,209 people, including women – which was a novelty at the time.

Every two years the subjects were brought in for weight and blood pressure measurements, questions and tests. Staff made daily visits to both Framingham hospitals to see who was ill, and chased death details through newspapers and coroners' reports.

Results poured out. Within a few years they had figures correlating heart disease with blood pressure, obesity and cholesterol. The age of risk factor minimisation was dawning. The doctors who argued high blood pressure was healthy, because it kept blood flowing through narrowed arteries, were silenced. By 1960 there was enough data to implicate smoking and diabetes. Since then it has generated over 2,000 papers, and a tsunami of information about diet, exercise and everything else that goes into keeping your blood vessels healthy.

Today everyone knows exercise and eating makes a big difference. It seems bizarre that there were ever well qualified sceptics to convince. An array of drugs exists to treat blood pressure and cholesterol, but the real legacy is a concept. Like gravity making apples fall, and the earth rotating the sun, it is obvious when the evidence is presented, but somebody had to think of it first. Heart disease is not fixed, and it is not inevitable. A large part of heart disease is behaviour. The same is true of other big-ticket diseases like cancer. Yes, inheritance – your personal genetic susceptibility – plays a significant part, but inheritance is the hand you are dealt. Behaviour is how you play it. Everything you have heard about healthy living arose because some people back in the 1940s thought that little town in New England should be investigated. You have never been told to live as you want because the future can't be changed. You have been told that your health future is dictated by what you do. You have been told that because of Framingham.

Just where the logic of healthy food leads is the next chapter in Framingham's legacy.

References

Bitton, A., & Gaziano, T. (2010). The Framingham Heart Study's Impact on Global Risk Assessment. *Progress in Cardiovascular Diseases*, 53(1), 68-78.

Bovenberg, J., Hansell, A., Hoogh, K., & Knoppers, B. (2015). Nature, nurture and exposure. *The EMBO Reports*, 16(4), 404-406.

Giroux (2013). The Framingham Study and the Constitution of a Restrictive Concept of Risk Factor. *Social History of Medicine*, 26(1), 94-112.

Greenberg, H. (2010). The Global Impact of the Framingham Heart Study. *Progress in Cardiovascular Diseases*, 53(1), 1-2.

Kreger, B. (1991). Coronary risk factors: Insights from Framingham. *Clinical Cardiology*, 14(S3), 3-12.

Mahmood, S.S., Levy, D., et al. (2014). The Framingham Heart Study and the Epidemiology of Cardiovascular Diseases: A Historical Perspective. *Lancet*, 383(9921): 999–1008.

Oppenheimer, G.M. (2005). Becoming the Framingham Study 1947 to 1950. *American Journal of Public Health*, 95(4).

Wilson, P. (2010). Preface—Global Impact of the Framingham Heart Study. *Progress in Cardiovascular Diseases*, 53(1).

www.cdc.gov/nchs/data/nvsr/nvsr61/nvsr61_07.pdf (last accessed November 2018)

5

PHARM FRESH EATING

Functional foods, super foods, nutraceuticals and bioactives

It appears Hippocrates did not say, 'Let food be thy medicine,' which is a pity;[1] everyone thinks he did and it is not a bad line. Regardless, the sentiment resonates. One of the biggest themes in the science of long life is the medicinal power of things edible.

When I was at medical school, in the 1980s, food was fuel. It was enough to eat sensibly: go easy on animal fat, lose some weight and don't take vitamins unless you are medically diagnosed as deficient. If it got more complex than that, you needed drugs. There was a lot of talking about drugs, and very little talking about food.[2] Food really only got attention on the rare occasions it caused serious pathology, like coeliac disease (where gluten attacks the bowel), and lactose intolerance (where the sugar lactose can't be digested).

The medical establishment did not deny the natural world contained molecules that affect metabolism such as aspirin, penicillin, and morphine.[3] In fact, doctors spent all day immersed in the subject. But they thought biologically active compounds should be stripped out of the plants they grew in, pressed into pills and swallowed in line

---

1 Adelman, J., & Haushofer, L. (2018). Introduction: Food as Medicine, Medicine as Food. *Journal of the History of Medicine and Allied Sciences*, 73(2), 127-134.
2 I do not recall a single lecture in the six-year degree about food.
3 Respectively, willow bark, mould and poppies.

with a prescription. That was the place for serious food chemistry: the substrate for drugs.

At the same time, the establishment also knew that certain patterns of eating were healthy. Or at least, I assume they knew. The literature on healthy eating has said for decades that coloured vegetables, fibre and sea food, for instance, are healthy things to eat, but that more than a little salt, alcohol and red meat are not. Presumably some doctors noticed, though it never figured in medical education or played much of a role in advice to patients. Medicine at the sharp end was about fixing things with surgery and exotic pharmaceuticals. What people had for dinner never got a look in.

Since the 1980s a different way of looking at the food and drug connection has been gaining ground. It first took root in Japan, and has since become an international industry, a huge focus for researchers and an imperative for people who want to maximise their health and longevity. The different way is functional food. There is no agreed definition but, in essence, it is a food, not a purified chemical, that delivers biologically active molecules over and above normal nutrition. That means a food that lowers cholesterol, or stabilises gut bacteria, or mops up free radicals. A related concept is nutraceutical, or nutrition-cum-pharmaceutical, which is the active fraction of functional food in concentrated form, like fish oil.

There are various synonyms – superfood for functional food, and bioactive for nutraceutical – but the concept is the same: food, or its immediate derivatives, with the kick of a drug.

There are many variations. In its simplest form, a functional food is a whole food with a naturally high level of biologically active constituents. Examples include herrings and pomegranate. Foods that are not traditional in the West, like quinoa and seaweed, are getting attention because of their potential in this regard.

The next step is food that is artificially tweaked. Farmers now breed cows that make one type of milk protein over another (A2 instead of A1), and feed hens with vitamins and healthy fats to fortify their eggs. Manufacturers offer spreads that lower cholesterol and hamburger patties with oat fibre. Not all these innovations are good ideas, but new thinking always has its baggage (see Spoiled for choice).

Inevitably, genetic modification has been recruited to the cause. Pink pineapples, red oranges,[4] high-fibre wheat, omega-3 canola oil and dozens more crops with a superfood twist are in the test field or on the market. Genetic modification used to be about the farmer's end of the equation: less pesticides and a longer shelf life. The technology is readily adapted to enriching plants, but the Faustian bargain involved has created an acute dilemma for marketing: the sort of consumers who would embrace the products are unlikely to embrace the concept behind them. So far, the companies involved have elected not to enthuse about their achievements publicly.

Then there are extracts. That refers to the bioactive component of a food split out on its own as a pill or a powder, which is useful where the benefit requires a higher intake than diet delivers. Herbs and spices can be maximised this way, as can dietary novelties like algae and olive leaves. Many very useful plants are difficult to eat outright, or to eat enough of, and the second half of the book describes a number of the notable ones. This is the world of supplements.

The goal is a slow accretion of physiological changes which, over years, keeps vital organs healthy. It is not radical in principle. Nobody disputes that heart disease and cancer come from gradual changes in our cells, or that the risk of acquiring them is affected by how you live your life. In particular, the risk is reduced by eating the right things,

---

4   For well-informed readers, I acknowledge there have always been blood oranges. But the natural kind need a frost to set whereas the GM version can be grown without one, and therefore much more widely.

and increased by eating the wrong ones. A wealth of evidence ties reduced risk to certain elements in healthy food, particularly plants (see <u>Nutraceuticals and where they come from</u>). It is a small step in logic to say that if plants rich in those elements, extracts of such plants, and extracts of similar compounds from other sources, form a regular part of one's daily intake they may focus the benefits of healthy food.

Incremental treatments are no stranger to mainstream medicine. Many people take pills to lower their blood pressure even though high blood pressure is not a disease and causes no symptoms. It is lowered to reduce the wear and tear on blood vessel walls which one day, after years, becomes a heart attack or stroke. The same principle applies to cholesterol: raised cholesterol is not a disease, but becomes one if left long enough. Drugs that lower cholesterol are the most widely prescribed in the world. So functional food is off to a good start: small daily changes matter.

However, the concept must compete in a crowded space. The public mind is saturated with diet advice of variable quality and contradictory principles: diets that reject meat, diets that emphasise meat, things that are bad for you (chocolate, wine, coffee), things that are good for you (chocolate, wine, coffee), and hundreds of variations that change with every headline. A new philosophy has to be heard above the noise. Functional food is an evolving idea but it rests on well-known patterns of healthy eating and the solid science that explains them. For decades researchers have sought out the diets around the planet that give health and long life, and analysed the elements within them that do the work. Functional food is the natural next step. Once you know what works, and we largely do, then the obvious imperative is to emphasise it.

References

Adelman, J., & Haushofer, L. (2018). Introduction: Food as Medicine, Medicine as Food. *Journal of the History of Medicine and Allied Sciences,* 73(2), 127-134.

Angiolillo, L., Conte, A., & Del Nobile, M. (2015). Technological strategies to produce functional meat burgers. *LWT - Food Science and Technology,* 62(1), 697-703.

Bigliardi, B., & Galati, F. (2013). Innovation trends in the food industry: The case of functional foods. *Trends in Food Science & Technology,* 31(2), 118-129.

Brooke-Taylor, S., Dwyer, K., Woodford, K., & Kost, N. (2017). Systematic Review of the Gastrointestinal Effects of A1 Compared with A2 β-Casein. *Advances in Nutrition,* 8(5), 739-748.

Corbo, M., Bevilacqua, A., Petruzzi, L., Casanova, F., & Sinigaglia, M. (2014). Functional Beverages: The Emerging Side of Functional Foods. *Comprehensive Reviews in Food Science and Food Safety,* 13(6), 1192-1206.

Farr, D. (1997). Functional foods. *Cancer Letters,* 114(1), 59-63.

István, S., Kápolna, E., Kápolna, B., & Lugasi, A. (2008). Functional food. Product development, marketing and consumer acceptance—A review. *Appetite,* 51(3), 456-467.

Jukema, J., Cannon, C., de Craen, A., et al. (2012). The Controversies of Statin Therapy. *Journal of the American Journal of Cardiology,* 60(10).

Le Page, M. (2018). A new kind of superfood. *New Scientist.*

Mohamed, S., et al., (2011). Seaweeds: A sustainable functional food for complementary and alternative therapy, *Trends in Food Science & Technology.*

Vel Szic, K.S., Declerck, K., Vidaković, M., & Vanden Berghe, W. (2015). From inflammaging to healthy aging by dietary lifestyle choices: is epigenetics the key to personalized nutrition? *Clinical Epigenetics,* 7(1).

6

NUTRACEUTICALS AND WHERE THEY COME FROM
What they are and why they work

The difference between food and drugs is, as we have seen, one of shades and nuances. What sits in no man's land are food molecules that go beyond ordinary nutrition. They are nutraceuticals. We eat them but we do not have to, although eating more of them appears to make us live longer. They are not essential like protein, carbohydrates and vitamins, but they grease the wheels of a very long existence on this earth just like drugs do. Seeking out these molecules, or seeking out the fraction of food that contains them, is a major strategy in the goal of living well for as long as possible.

The concept of a nutraceutical is a loose one and difficulties with classification abound. For instance, is alcohol a nutraceutical? A lot of brewers and vintners would like you to think so, but there is no consensus on the benefit of alcohol compared to its considerable harm.

Leaving the fringes alone, most of the quality nutraceutical research concerns the health giving, anti-ageing, antioxidant and anti-inflammatory properties of *phytochemicals*, which means chemicals from plants. Although the field does not belong to phytochemicals exclusively – fats from fish are nutraceuticals, for instance – they dominate.[1]

---

1 As discussed in <u>Omega-3 or not Omega-3: That is the question</u>, even the omega-3 in fish comes from algae at the bottom of the food chain.

Strictly speaking, a phytochemical is any chemical from a plant (*phyto* meaning 'plant' in Greek). In practice, the term is used for the health-giving ones, and humanity has a long history of exploiting them. They were the sole source of medicine before industrial chemistry took over, and even today around a quarter of prescription drugs have a plant ingredient.

Plants make phytochemicals for various reasons, like attracting bees, but the main reason is defence. Phytochemicals heal wounds, kill bacteria (which gives us antibiotics) and absorb UV light. They often show themselves as vibrant colours, particularly the light absorbers, which is why it is healthy to eat a rainbow.[2]

Phytochemicals also arise from stress. When a plant has too much heat or too little water, for instance, it adapts: deeper roots, smaller pores, more purple sun-soaking pigment. Distressed plants emit breeze-borne chemicals to warn the neighbours. The survival programme is coordinated by free radicals, those unstable, firecracker molecules described in The inflammage. Free radicals are friend and foe: they deliver key signals but damage everything they bang into. Why plant life conferred such an important job on such unsuitable candidates is not clear, but it did, and plants have relied on antioxidant phytochemicals ever since to contain the free radicals and limit the harm. So stress means both more free radicals and more phyto–chemicals to corral them to just where they are needed.

And phytochemicals taste funny. Plants have been fending off things that want to eat them ever since they encountered insects, and the game is well advanced. Nettles sting and peppers burn because the plant wants to be left alone and numerous other chemicals, distasteful to browsers, permeate the plant kingdom and therefore the domestic

---

2   One of the reasons berries are so healthy is that they have a high ratio of surface to volume, and hence high levels of light-protecting, polyphenol pigments like anthocyanins that sit in the skin.

34

hearth. The pungency of cloves and mustard, the tang of mint, the warmth of nutmeg and scores of other kitchen staples are the fallout from this arms race. It is interesting to realise, next time you add spice to something, that the flavour was supposed to be repellent. (I emphasise, as above, in case it appears plants have shot themselves in the foot over this, that the traditional enemy was insects, not people.)

So phytochemicals are multipronged threat managers whose properties translate, by fortunate serendipity, to well-being in humans. Fruit and vegetables have them in abundance, but so do grains, nuts, dark chocolate, spices, herbs, and tea and coffee along with novel sources such as olive leaves and tree sap.

At this juncture a modicum of chemistry is helpful, if you can bear with me. There are thousands of phytochemicals, but their basic units are remarkably consistent. Most are phenols, or phenol aggregates. A *phenol* is a ring of six carbon atoms with certain side arms, and polyphenols are molecules made of these rings stuck together in various ways, like LEGO®.[3] Resveratrol (grapes), curcumin (turmeric) and catechins (tea), discussed in the chapters to come, are all built this way, as are many others. The phenomenon reflects efficiency: like car factories, production lines in plants are most productive making products they recognise.

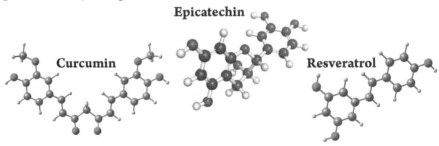

Epicatechin

Curcumin

Resveratrol

---

3   Some molecules of interest are single rings, but in the interests of conciseness, the term polyphenol is often used to cover both types.

Why they should work for us is a head scratcher. It is very nice of plants to medicate us as well as feed us, but it is not obvious why they do it. Maybe it is coincidence; plants make so many different molecules a few are bound to interact with animal metabolism.

More intriguingly, it may be that animals piggyback on useful clues about the environment. If some polyphenols mean drought, for instance, animals who live in the same location notice, at a molecular level, what the plants they eat are 'saying', and adapt.

And maybe they poison us. Noxious chemicals stop insects eating plants and when we eat the same plants, we get a little dose too. A little dose of poison stirs up cell repair mechanisms. As stated, cell repair sags as you get older. Keeping cells patched up and working is the central tenet of healthy ageing, so stimulating the maintenance teams does more good than harm.

Biologists call this *hormesis*. That is, the principle that a small dose of something toxic is healthy. It works like the fire brigade. If the fire brigade gets called once a week it will be a disciplined force. But if calls never come, the members will forget what to do. This is why stresses like exercise and calorie restriction are healthy: controlled shocks turn on protective reactions. Even radiation, in tiny doses, promotes a longer life.

Hormesis might explain alcohol. As mentioned, alcohol's properties are debated with vigour. Large population studies purport to show very modest drinking is healthy, but many experts do not concur and point to alcohol's toxicity. Maybe they are wrong for the right reasons: toxicity is the point. In strict moderation.

Curcumin and resveratrol, two of the standout anti-ageing molecules, activate stress response pathways, and an expanding list of plant substances is joining them. It is odd to think the vital parts of fruit and vegetables work in part by selective poisoning, but increasing evidence suggests it is so. As the saying goes, 'What does not kill you makes you stronger' and plants have been doing it to us for millennia.

References

Adnani, N., Rajski, S.R., & Bugni, T.S. (2017). Symbiosis-inspired approaches to antibiotic discovery. *Natural Product Reports, 34*(7), 784-814.

Agati, G., Azzarello, E., Pollastri, S., & Tattini, M. (2012). Flavonoids as antioxidants in plants: Location and functional significance. *Plant Science, 196,* 67-76.

Ann Lila, M. (2006). The nature versus nurture debate on bioactive phytochemicals: the genome versus terroir. *Journal of the Science of Food and Agriculture, 86*(15), 2510-2515.

Bandurska, H., Niedziela, J., & Chadzinikolau, T. (2013). Separate and combined responses to water deficit and UV-B radiation. *Plant Science, 213,* 98-105.

Birringer, M. (2011). Hormetics: Dietary Triggers of an Adaptive Stress Response. *Pharmaceutical Research, 28*(11), 2680-2694.

Calabrese, V., Cornelius, C., Dinkova Kostova, A., & Calabrese, E. (2009). Vitagenes, cellular stress response, and acetylcarnitine: Relevance to hormesis. *BioFactors (Electronic), 35*(2), 146-160.

Capanoglu, E. (2010). The potential of priming in food production. *Trends in Food Science & Technology, 21*(8), 399-407.

Cespedes, C., Aqueveque, P., Avila, J., Alarcon, J., & Kubo, I. (2015). New advances in chemical defenses of plants: researches in calceolariaceae. *Phytochemistry Reviews, 14*(3), 367-380.

De Gara, L., Locato, V., Dipierro, S., & de Pinto, M. (2010). Redox homeostasis in plants. The challenge of living with endogenous oxygen production. *Respiratory Physiology & Neurobiology, 173,* S13-S19.

Del Rio, D., Rodriguez-Mateos, A., Spencer, J.P.E, Tognolini, M., Borges, G., & Crozier, A. (2013). Dietary (Poly)phenolics in Human Health: Structures, Bioavailability, and Evidence of Protective Effects Against Chronic Diseases. *Antioxidants & Redox Signaling, 18*(14), 1818-1892.

El Gharras, H. (2009). Polyphenols: food sources, properties and applications – a review. *International Journal of Food Science & Technology, 44*(12).

Gaascht, F., Dicato, M., & Diederich, M. (2015). Coffee provides a natural multitarget pharmacopeia against the hallmarks of cancer. *Genes & Nutrition, 10*(6), 1-17.

Gaman, L., Stoian, I., & Atanasiu, V. (2011). Can ageing be slowed?: Hormetic and redox perspectives. *Journal of Medicine and Life, 4*(4), 346-351.

Hatier, J., & Gould, K. (2008). Foliar anthocyanins as modulators of stress signals. *Journal of Theoretical Biology, 253*(3), 625-627.

Howitz, K.T., & Sinclair, D.A. (2008). Xenohormesis: Sensing the Chemical Cues of Other Species. *Cell, 133*(3), 387-391.

Ismail, T. (2017). Emerging roles for ROS and RNS – versatile molecules in plants. *Journal of Experimental Botany, 68*(16), 4413–4416.

Khoo, H.-E., Prasad, K.N., Kong, K.-W., Jiang, Y., & Ismail, A. (2011). Carotenoids and Their Isomers: Color Pigments in Fruits and Vegetables. *Molecules,* 16, 1710-1738.

Kim, J., Lee, H. J. and Lee, K. W. (2010). Naturally occurring phytochemicals for the prevention of Alzheimer's disease. *Journal of Neurochemistry,* 112, 1415–1430.

Lamming, D., Wood, J., & Sinclair, D. (2004). MicroReview: Small molecules that regulate lifespan: evidence for xenohormesis. *Molecular Microbiology,* 53(4).

Lampe, J. (2003). Spicing up a vegetarian diet: chemopreventive effects of phytochemicals. *The American Journal of Clinical Nutrition,* 78(3) 579S-583S.

Mattson, M.P. (2008). Dietary Factors, Hormesis and Health. *Ageing Research Reviews,* 7(1), 43-48.

Matsumoto, C., Miedema, M.D., Ofman, P., Gaziano,J.M., & Sesso, H.D. (2014). An expanding knowledge of the mechanisms and effects of alcohol consumption on cardiovascular disease. *Journal of Cardiopulmonary Rehabilitation and Prevention,* 34(3), 159-71.

Menendez, J.A., Joven, J., Aragonès, G, et al. (2013). Xenohormetic and anti-aging activity of secoiridoid polyphenols present in extra virgin olive oil: A new family of gerosuppressant agents. *Cell Cycle,* 12(4), 555-578.

Murugaiyah, V., & Mattson, M. (2015). Neurohormetic phytochemicals: An evolutionary–bioenergetic perspective. *Neurochemistry International,* 89, 271-280.

Rattan, S. (2008). Hormesis in aging. *Ageing Research Reviews,* 7(1), 63-78.

Si, H., & Liu, D. (2014). Dietary antiaging phytochemicals and mechanisms associated with prolonged survival. *The Journal of Nutritional Biochemistry,* 25(6), 581-591.

Son, T., Camandola, S., & Mattson, M. (2008). Hormetic Dietary Phytochemicals. *NeuroMolecular Medicine,* 10(4), 236-246.

Tresserra-Rimbau, A., Lamuela-Raventos, R.M., Moreno, J.J. (2018). Polyphenols, food and pharma. Current knowledge and directions for future research. *Biochemical Pharmacology,* 156, 186-195.

Vaiserman, A. (2011). Hormesis and epigenetics: Is there a link? *Ageing Research Reviews,* 10(4), 413-421.

Weichselbaum, E., & Buttriss, J. (2010). Polyphenols in the diet. *Nutrition Bulletin,* 35(2).

Yin, X., Singer, S.D., Qiao, H., et al. (2016). Insights into the Mechanisms Underlying Ultraviolet-C Induced Resveratrol Metabolism in Grapevine (V. amurensisRupr.) cv. "Tonghua-3." *Frontiers in Plant Science,* 7(503).

Zahedi, R., & Sickmann, A. (2013). Plant proteins under oxidative attack. *Proteomics,* 13(6), 932-940.

Zenkov, N., Chechushkov, A., Kozhin, P., Kandalintseva, N., Martinovich, G., & Menshchikova, E. (2016). Plant phenols and autophagy. *Biochemistry (Moscow),* 81(4), 297-314.

Current Pharmaceutical Biotechnology, (2016). Editorial Phytochemicals for Human Diseases: An Update. 17(11).

7

EPIGENETICS AND FOOD
AS INFORMATION
Food that writes your software

Our body parts start, like all complex objects, with a blueprint. The Eiffel Tower and the Golden Gate Bridge were not bolted together with random pieces, and neither are you. Ever since the 1950s we have known that the plans for living things are long molecules of deoxyribonucleic acid, or DNA, which functions like Morse code. There are four units in the sequence, not two, but the principle is the same: a line of symbols that codes a message. A length of DNA that describes a specific thing like the colour of your eyes is a gene. A collection of genes, around two metres of DNA, describes an organism. Genes are also useful for sorting out who your relatives are and catching criminals.

However, a blueprint needs someone to open it up and put together the pieces it describes. Similarly, cells have a machinery of proteins that build new structures and what they make depends on the DNA they read. Your DNA code is fixed and every cell has the same copy, so brain cells, bone cells and blood cells vary only because they were assembled from different pages of the instruction book. Reading genes doesn't just direct the right cells to grow in the right places, it manipulates how they live, work and die. That means health and longevity. Turns out, the way genes are read has a lot to do with the world you live in—the stress you feel, the exercise you take, the cigarettes you smoke and, in particular, the food you eat turns genes on and off like light bulbs.

To cite a dramatic example, queens and workers in a beehive have the same DNA, but they turn out differently because royal jelly, which selected grubs are reared on, turns off the genes that make worker bees and turns on the ones that make queens.

It works because DNA can be modified, without changing the code sequence, to switch the reading on and off. Scientists call this *epigenetics* (epi is Greek for 'on'). The prime mechanism, called *methylation*, occurs when a molecule called a methyl group is stuck into the DNA sequence like a pin so reading proteins can't latch on. As you get older, most of your genes wind up with less methylation, although some get more, and the imbalance has a lot to do with age-related diseases like cancer and frailty in general. A stand-out factor that appears responsible is the chronic inflammation that age brings (see The inflammage), as inflamed tissue has more methylation points.

It also seems plausible – the jury has not returned yet – that this is a major route for the well-known effect of diet on big ageing diseases like cancer. The wrong food stirs up inflammation which creates a chain which links diet, chronic inflammation and pathological methylation changes.

Epigenetics also features at the other end of life. Babies of underfed mothers are more likely to be obese when they are adults as if they were programmed in the womb to compensate for their environment. They can even pass it on. Dutch war babies in the mid-1940s were small and sickly but, so in turn, were their own children who were born in normal times, and DNA methylation appears to be responsible. Methylation is a complex subject, but it may connect the dots between adversity in early life, or of social deprivation generally, and illness as an adult.

It also connects the dots between illness and food. Fascinating clues are also emerging that substances as diverse as pesticides and chemotherapy drugs might cause epigenetic changes that subsequent generations inherit.

Plant polyphenols can alter DNA methylation; they can also manipulate *histone modification*, another epigenetic mechanism which controls the way DNA is coiled and uncoiled so the reading machine can get at it. Dietary elements that can do these tricks include soy beans, resveratrol, curcumin, green tea, coffee, cruciferous vegetables and garlic.

The power of healthy food, particularly plant polyphenols, to modify your epigenetic state is a new and developing field, but enough is known to say that food is not just fuel and building blocks. Food is instructions. Food changes you. To put the issue into the digital age, food is information.

A closely related concept concerns the gene readers themselves, which nutraceuticals can interfere with. As mentioned in The inflammage, the NF-kB protein is a key bottleneck in the inflammation cascade, which controls whether 400 or so genes that code for inflammatory proteins are read. Obstructing NF-kB shuts down the factory, and is a common tactic of nutraceuticals like curcumin and epigallocatechin-3-gallate (EGCG) from tea.

A related protein is SIRT1, the most prominent member of a group of enzymes called *sirtuins*, or Silent Information Regulators, which have a lot to do with how well and how quickly living things age. SIRT1 has a multipronged effect on gene reading, which modulates inflammation, cell survival and oxidative balance (see The inflammage).

It also drives the longevity-inducing technique of calorie restriction. It is well known (but hard to put into practice), that eating less while consuming essential nutrition is a potent way of lengthening life and fending off age-related diseases like cancer and diabetes. Calorie restriction causes laboratory animals to live longer. It is a feature of long-lived communities like those on Okinawa in Japan. People living in Denmark and Norway during wartime who managed, against the odds, to eat a balanced diet while eating less dramatically reduced their incidence of heart disease and early death. Multiple metabolic pathways contribute, but the major benefit seems to come from stimulating SIRT1. SIRT1 is also stimulated by exercise, and suppressed by sugar and fat. It is potently activated by resveratrol, one of the main polyphenols in grapes, particularly their seeds, as well as a variety of other plants like gingko biloba, onions (quercetin), black currants, persimmons and cocoa.

There are many other complex enzyme systems in play, and details are being hunted down in laboratories across the globe, but the point is that the sort of food you should be eating shuts down inflammation in the control room. It is food that says 'shhhh'; food that tames the dragon. It writes your programme, and your life and health ride on being programmed correctly.

References

Ahmed, F. (2010). Epigenetics: Tales of adversity. *Nature, 468*(7327), S20-S20.

Ahn, K.S., & Aggarwal, B.B. (2005). Transcription factor NF-kappaB: a sensor for smoke and stress signals. *Annals of the New York Academy of Sciences,* 1056, 218-233.

Ayissi, V., Ebrahimi, A., & Schluesenner, H. (2014). Epigenetic effects of natural polyphenols: A focus on SIRT1-mediated mechanisms. *Molecular Nutrition & Food Research, 58*(1), 22-32.

Bhullar, K., & Hubbard, B. (2015). Lifespan and healthspan extension by resveratrol. *Biochimica et Biophysica Acta (BBA) - Molecular Basis of Disease,* 1852(6), 1209-1218.

Chango, A., & Pogribny, I.P. (2015). Considering Maternal Dietary Modulators for Epigenetic Regulation and Programming of the Fetal Epigenome. *Nutrients, 7*(4), 2748-2770.

Choi, S., & Friso, S. (2010). Epigenetics: A New Bridge between Nutrition and Health. *Advances in Nutrition,* 1(1), 8-16.

Christodoulou, M., Thomas, A., Poulain, S., Vidakovic, M., Lahtela-Kakkonen, M., Matulis, D., Bertrand, P., Bartova, E., Blanquart, C., Mikros, E., Fokialakis, N., Passarella, D., Benhida, R., & Martinet, N. (2014). Can we use the epigenetic bioactivity of caloric restriction and phytochemicals to promote healthy ageing? *MedChemComm*, 5(12), 1804-1820.

Chu, Y., Wise, M., Gulvady, A., Chang, T., Kendra, D., Jan-Willem van Klinken, B., Shi, Y., & O'Shea, M. (2013). In vitro antioxidant capacity and anti-inflammatory activity of seven common oats. *Food Chemistry*, 139(1), 426-431.

Cuevas, A., Saavedra, N., Salazar, L., & Abdalla, D. (2013). Modulation of Immune Function by Polyphenols: Possible Contribution of Epigenetic Factors. *Nutrients*, 5(7), 2314-2332.

Das, S., Balasubramanian, P., & Weerasekara, Y. (2017). Nutrition modulation of human aging: The calorie restriction paradigm. *Molecular and Cellular Endocrinology*, 455, 148-157.

Dolinsky, V., & Dyck, J. (2011). Calorie restriction and resveratrol in cardiovascular health and disease. *Biochimica et Biophysica Acta (BBA) - Molecular Basis of Disease*, 1812(11), 1477-1489.

Elizabeth A. Mazzio, K. (2014). Epigenetics and Nutritional Environmental Signals. *Integrative and Comparative Biology*, 54(1).

Gescher, A. (2013). Curcumin as a regulator of epigenetic events. *Molecular Nutrition & Food Research*, 57(9), 1619-1629.

Guerrero-Bosagna, C.M., & Skinner, M.K. (2014). Environmental epigenetics and phytoestrogen/phytochemical exposures. *The Journal of Steroid Biochemistry and Molecular Biology*, 139, 270-276.

Inbar-Feigenberg, M, et al. Basic concepts of epigenetics. *Fertility and Sterility*, 99(3), 607 – 615.

Kappil, M., Wright, R.O., & Sanders, A.P. (2016). Developmental Origins of Common Disease: Epigenetic Contributions to Obesity. *Annual Review of Genomics and Human Genetics*, 17, 177-192.

Kaushik, P., & Anderson, J. (2016). Obesity: epigenetic aspects. *Biomolecular Concepts*, 7(3).

Kim, J., Chen, J., & Lou, Z. (2008). DBC1 is a negative regulator of SIRT1. *Nature*, 451(7178), 583-586.

Knutson, M., & Leeuwenburgh, C. (2008). Resveratrol and novel potent activators of Sirt1: effects on aging and age-related diseases. *Nutrition Reviews*, 66(10), 591-596.

López-Lluch, G., & Navas, P. (2016). Calorie restriction as an intervention in ageing. *The Journal of Physiology*, 594(8), 2043-2060.

Malcomson, F., & Mathers, J. (2017). Nutrition, epigenetics and health through life. *Nutrition Bulletin*, 42(3), 254-265.

Marques, F., Markus, M., & Morris, B. (2009). Resveratrol: Cellular actions of a potent natural chemical that confers a diversity of health benefits. *The International Journal of Biochemistry & Cell Biology*, 41(11), 2125-2128.

McKay, J., & Mathers, J. (2011). Diet induced epigenetic changes and their implications for health. *Acta Physiologica*, 202(2).

Mead, M.N. (2007). Nutrigenomics: The Genome–Food Interface. *Environmental Health Perspectives*, 115(12), A582-A589.

Most, J., Tosti, V., Redman, L., & Fontana, L. (2017). Calorie restriction in humans: An update. *Ageing Research Reviews*, 39, 36-45.

Mulligan, C. (2016). Early Environments, Stress, and the Epigenetics of Human Health. *Annual Review of Anthropology*, 45, 233-249.

Muriach, M., Flores-Bellver, M., Romero, F., & Barcia, J. (2014). Diabetes and the Brain: Oxidative Stress, Inflammation, and Autophagy. *Oxidative Medicine and Cellular Longevity.*

Peterson, C., & Laniel, M. (2004). Histones and histone modifications. *Current Biology*, 14(14), R546-R551.

Petersen, K., & Smith, C. (2016). Ageing-Associated Oxidative Stress and Inflammation Are Alleviated by Products from Grapes. *Oxidative Medicine and Cellular Longevity.*

Rabadán-Chávez, G., Miliar Garcia, A., Paniagua Castro, N., Escalona Cardoso, G., Quevedo-Corona, L., Reyes-Maldonado, E., & Jaramillo-Flores, M. (2016). Modulating the expression of genes associated with hepatic lipid metabolism, lipoperoxidation and inflammation by cocoa, cocoa extract and cocoa flavanols related to hepatic steatosis induced by a hypercaloric diet. *Food Research International*, 89, 937-945.

Remely, M., Lovrecic, L., Garza, A., Migliore, L., Peterlin, B., Milagro, F., Martinez, A., & Haslberger, A. (2015). Therapeutic perspectives of epigenetically active nutrients. *British Journal of Pharmacology*, 172(11), 2756-2768.

Reuter, S., Gupta, S., Park, B., Goel, A., & Aggarwal, B. (2011). Epigenetic changes induced by curcumin and other natural compounds. *Genes & Nutrition*, 6(2), 93-108.

Sapienza, C., & Issa, J. (2016). Diet, Nutrition, and Cancer Epigenetics. *Annual Review of Nutrition*, 36, 665-681.

Setchell, K. (2017). The history and basic science development of soy isoflavones. *Menopause*, 24(12), 1338-1350.

Shimizu, M. Multifunctions of dietary polyphenols in the regulation of intestinal inflammation. *Journal of Food and Drug Analysis*, 25(1), 93 – 99.

Shukla, S., Meeran, S., & Katiyar, S. (2014). Epigenetic regulation by selected dietary phytochemicals in cancer chemoprevention. *Cancer Letters*, 355(1), 9-17.

Singh, B., Singh, H., Singh, A., Naqvi, A., & Singh, B. (2014). Dietary phytochemicals alter epigenetic events and signaling pathways for inhibition of metastasis cascade. *Cancer and Metastasis Reviews*, 33(1), 41-85.

Spannhoff, A., Kim, Y., Raynal, N., Gharibyan, V., Su, M., Zhou, Y., Li, J., Castellano, S., Sbardella, G., Issa, J., & Bedford, M. (2011). Histone deacetylase inhibitor activity in royal jelly might facilitate caste switching in bees. *The EMBO Reports*, 12(3), 238-243.

Stringhini, S (2015). Life-course socioeconomic status and DNA methylation of genes regulating inflammation. *International Journal of Epidemiology*, 44(4),

Stefanska, B., & MacEwan, D. (2015). Epigenetics and pharmacology. *British Journal of Pharmacology*, 172(11), 2701-2704.

Tang, B. (2016). Sirt1 and the Mitochondria. *Molecules and Cells*, 39(2), 87-95.

Tousoulis, D., Psarros, C., Demosthenous, M., Patel, R., Antoniades, C., & Stefanadis, C. (2014). Innate and Adaptive Inflammation as a Therapeutic Target in Vascular Disease. *Journal of the American College of Cardiology,* 63(23), 2491-2502.

Vaiserman, A. (2011). Hormesis and epigenetics: Is there a link? *Ageing Research Reviews,* 10(4), 413-421.

Wong, S., & Tang, B. (2016). SIRT1 as a therapeutic target for Alzheimer's disease. *Reviews in the Neurosciences,* 27(8), 813-825.

Zhang, J., Rane, G., Dai, X., Shanmugam, M., Arfuso, F., Samy, R., Lai, M., Kappei, D., Kumar, A., & Sethi, G. (2016). Ageing and the telomere connection: An intimate relationship with inflammation. *Ageing Research Reviews,* 25, 55-69.

Zinovkina, L., & Zinovkin, R. (2015). DNA methylation, mitochondria, and programmed aging. *Biochemistry (Moscow),* 80(12), 1571-1577.

8

THE ORCHESTRA, NOT THE SOLOIST
Effective supplements work as a team

The idea that free radicals, the natural byproducts of burning food, might be central to ageing, as per The inflammage, was sprung on the world in 1956 by a researcher called Denham Harman.[1] His insight, like all good ones, was both ground-breaking and simple. Everything gets frail when it is old, so the explanation had to be universal. Free radicals are ubiquitous, yet dangerous and could be expected, via their unstable unpaired electrons, to attack the cells that made them. Damaged cells mean frailty, disease and death. Free radicals are neutralised by antioxidants, so the theory explained why people who eat lots of antioxidants – the Mediterranean diet, for instance – live longer and do not get the big diseases as often. It also explained why animals with low metabolic rates which burn proportionately less food live longer than those with high rates which burn more (elephants compared to hummingbirds). Everything added up.

Even better, particularly for the industrial food world, was the implication: take out the antioxidant bit and repackage it. Certain vitamins – like C, E and A – are potent antioxidants and come from plant food. Maybe they explained the longevity payoff from healthy

---

1   Harman, D. (1956). Aging: a theory based on free radical and radiation chemistry. *Journals of Gerontology*, 11:298-300.

eating. It was a call to action: eat more vitamins and live longer! It also excited investors. Never mind apples and carrots, get chemists to brew up the useful bit, pop it in a pill, and there you are. Instant longevity without the inconvenience of eating properly. Simple message, cheap ingredients and a public health winner. Since then, multivitamin pills have been the heart of the world supplement industry, relied on by millions to deliver a healthy metabolic balance.

Unfortunately, it hasn't worked. The world would be a rosier place if the premise was true, so a lot of attention has been paid to studying it. Factories have been pumping out vitamin pills for decades, so the information is out there. The large studies are in. The consensus is for failure. Taking vitamins in purified form does not make you live longer.

There is still a niche for people with deficiencies, of course. Vitamins are critical, and some experts argue mild deficiencies are common. The Western world is drowning in food, but too many rely on the highly processed kind and, for such people, vitamin supplements might be useful. There are also special situations, like vitamin D for frail elderly,[2] and folic acid (a B vitamin) for pregnant women. But beyond deficiency or special needs, pure substances falter. Simply put, if you are eating properly, synthetic vitamins are a waste of time.

However, there is no doubt vitamin-rich food is effective, and the evidence continues to accumulate. Living longer, staying healthier, keeping your heart and brain ticking, and fending off cancer are still rooted in eating a comprehensive range of plant food. That part of the theory is unassailable.

So what is going on? Are we concentrating on the wrong thing? Good food has thousands of candidates for the real source of longevity, so is some other chemical X the silver bullet?

---

2   I acknowledge, for the sake of completeness, there is ongoing research and debate about whether vitamin D supplementation could be useful for others too.

Far more likely, and widely accepted by experts, is that nothing works by itself. The evidence connects benefit with bioactives in food, not bioactives in a purified form. Food is an orchestra, a many-splendoured thing (as Shakespeare might have put it if he had been a food writer), which only works when multiple ingredients all pull together. It is a witches' brew of molecules which even chemists do not understand, but which only work their magic collectively. The pendulum doesn't work without the clock. It is a recurring theme in functional food, that food as nature made it is better than the individual parts, including those parts that seem to be most useful. It is possible they aren't the most useful at all, but much more likely they are cogs in a delicate piece of machinery and only function in unison.

This is not to criticise the idea of dietary supplements. Supplements are eminently credible if they retain the chemical complexity of a natural source, like turmeric or fish oil, or freeze-dried plant bits (grape seeds, for instance). The whole theme of this book is that complex anti-inflammatory supplements are worth taking. The problem lies with supplements of pure chemicals like resveratrol, not supplementation per se.

It comes back to our design. We have been formed to respond in subtle and multilayered ways to eating complex ingredients and, until the modern world, we knew nothing else. Humans are not petrol engines. Pure-form supplements are messing with the system.

Also, we are not identical. People differ widely in their genes, the complement of bugs in their bowel, and the myriad of enzymes and cells that create an individual metabolism. Even if a pure-form molecule improved the health of some people, which is unlikely, it would only be for those who won the lottery of coincidence that meshed it with their personal machinery; it would not be universal.

And one last thing … isolating a single molecule to make it more potent also makes it more toxic. Too much of a vitamin is poisonous and, although uncommon, cases of people making themselves ill on vitamins, particularly A, E and D, appear regularly in medical literature. Even more sinister is the evidence that ill effects are not limited to acute poisoning. Large studies have shown some pure-form supplements may subtly undermine your health and shorten your life if you take them when you did not need to. Examples include iron,[3] beta-carotene (a vitamin A precursor), selenium and vitamin E.

Supplements that work best and harm least come from food, or something closely related to it. The point is not whether it comes as a pill or freeze-dried powder, because useful things may well do. The point is whether it is a single substance, or a derivative that retains the complexity conferred by nature.

References

Assmann, G., Buono, P., Daniele, A., Della Valle, E., Farinaro, E., Ferns, G., Krogh, V., Kromhout, D., Masana, L., Merino, J., Misciagna, G., Panico, S., Riccardi, G., Rivellese, A., Rozza, F., Salvatore, F., Salvatore, V., Stranges, S., Trevisan, M., Trimarco, B., & Vetrani, C. (2014). Functional foods and cardiometabolic diseases. *Nutrition, Metabolism and Cardiovascular Diseases*, 24(12), 1272-1300.

Bjelakovic, G., Nikolova, D., & Gluud, C. (2013). Antioxidant Supplements to Prevent Mortality. *JAMA*, 310(11), 1178-1179.

Birringer, M. (2011). Hormetics: Dietary Triggers of an Adaptive Stress Response. *Pharmaceutical Research*, 28(11), 2680-2694.

Brandt, K., Christensen, L., Hansen-Møller, J., Hansen, S., Haraldsdottir, J., Jespersen, L., Purup, S., Kharazmi, A., Barkholt, V., Frøkiær, H., & Kobæk-Larsen, M. (2004). Health promoting compounds in vegetables and fruits. *Trends in Food Science & Technology*, 15(7), 384-393.

El Gharras, H. (2009). Polyphenols: food sources, properties and applications – a review. *International Journal of Food Science & Technology*, 44(12).

---

3   Iron is interesting. As per Bioavailability: Getting past the border guards, only one short section of the human bowel can absorb it. Although it is vital for our health, it appears there is little room for error in absorbing too much, and we have evolved to absorb minimal amounts even to the point that deficiencies are common.

Harman, D. (1956). Aging: a theory based on free radical and radiation chemistry. *The Journals of Gerontology,* 11:298-300.

Khurana, S., Venkataraman, K., Hollingsworth, A., Piche, M., & Tai, T. (2013). Polyphenols: Benefits to the Cardiovascular System in Health and in Aging. *Nutrients,* 5(10), 3779-3827.

Lichtenberg, D., & Pinchuk, I. (2015). Oxidative stress, the term and the concept. *Biochemical and Biophysical Research Communications,* 461(3), 441-444.

Liu, R.H. (2013). Health-Promoting Components of Fruits and Vegetables in the Diet. *Advances in Nutrition,* 4(3), 384S-392S.

Mithen, F.R.A.T.H.M. (2011). Plant Science and Human Nutrition: *Challenges in Assessing Health-Promoting Properties of Phytochemicals,* 23(7), 2483.

Moyer, M. (2014). Nutrition: Vitamins on trial. *Nature,* 510(7506), 462-464.

Paganini-Hill, A., Kawas, C.H, (2015). Corrada MM. Antioxidant Vitamin Intake and Mortality: The Leisure World Cohort Study. *American Journal of Epidemiology,* 181(2), 120-126.

Persson, P., & Persson, A. (2017). Vitamin supplementation. *Acta Physiologica,* 219(3), 537-539.

Prentice, A.M., Mendoza, Y.A., Pereira, D., et al. (2017). Dietary strategies for improving iron status: balancing safety and efficacy. *Nutrition Reviews,* 75(1), 49-60.

Russo, G., Tedesco, I., Spagnuolo, C., & Russo, M. (2017). Antioxidant polyphenols in cancer treatment: Friend, foe or foil? *Seminars in Cancer Biology,* 46, 1-13.

Rutkowski, M., & Grzegorczyk, K. (2012). Adverse effects of antioxidative vitamins. *International Journal of Occupational Medicine and Environmental Health,* 25(2), 105–121.

Sadowska-Bartosz, I., & Bartosz, G. (2014). Effect of Antioxidants Supplementation on Aging and Longevity. *BioMed Research International.*

Sesso, H., Christen, W., Bubes, V., Smith, J., MacFadyen, J., Schvartz, M., Manson, J., Glynn, R., Buring, J., & Gaziano, J. (2012). Multivitamins in the Prevention of Cardiovascular Disease in Men. *JAMA,* 308(17), 1751-1760.

Tresserra-Rimbau, A., Lamuela-Raventos, R.M., Moreno, J.J. (2018). Polyphenols, food and pharma. Current knowledge and directions for future research. *Biochemical Pharmacology,* 156, 186-195.

Ulbricht, C., & Chao, W. (2010). Phytochemicals in the Oncology Setting. *Current Treatment Options in Oncology,* 11(3), 95-10.

Ward, J. (2012). Should Antioxidant Vitamins be Routinely Recommended for Older People? *Drugs & Aging,* 12(3), 169-175.

Weinberg, E.D. Is addition of iron to processed foods safe for iron replete consumers? *Medical Hypotheses,* 73(6), 948 – 949

9

THE PROOF OF THE PUDDING

What to do about proof,
from a doctor who washed his hands

So... it is a cute idea. The theories are brilliant. The insights are extensive. But do functional food and nutraceuticals work? Is there proof?

Functional food is a smorgasbord, not a single drug, and extracting hard data is not straightforward. The natural world is complex. There are thousands of substances in any piece of plant or animal that can be eaten, and they spark thousands upon thousands of reactions inside your body.[1]

Functional food shows promise in the laboratory, but there is a gulf between lab rats and humans, particularly when the effects take years. True proof can only come from following people who eat something, then comparing their health with an equivalent group who do not. The technical challenges are huge. Such studies need large groups to be followed for years, if not decades, and they need to isolate the test item from everything else in each subject's lifestyle. Even when studies like this are done, experts argue about what they mean, particularly because of the last factor: the presence or absence of a positive result can always be blamed on something else. Maybe red wine appears

---

1 The typical diet contains 25,000 bioactive ingredients according to one authority. See Rajendran, P., Nandakumar, N., Rengarajan, T., Palaniswami, R., Gnanadhas, E., Lakshminarasaiah … Nishigaki, I. (2014). Antioxidants and human diseases. *Clinica Chimica Acta*, 436, 332–347. Pg 335.

healthy because it is a middle class tipple, consumed by people who tend to eat well and go to the gym. Maybe the trials that link coffee with heart attacks did not notice the subjects who enjoyed a cigarette with their morning cup. Maybe studies that pan vitamins are just badly designed. This is why big diet controversies, like alcohol and animal fat, never get sorted out. There is always room for argument.

There is also a challenge with cost. Drugs are tested in big studies because they are patented, and make money (and lots of it) if they work. Food is common property, and benefits proven can be picked up by everyone in the industry. The business case for dropping millions in efficacy studies is much harder to make.

Many people, particularly professional advisers, think the hurdles are enough reason to leave the issue alone. Officialdom is conservative, and does not like to put its stamp on anything until the benefits are thoroughly pinned down. Until the mainstream scientists line up, they prefer to sit on their hands, which means bureaucrats operate well behind the horizons researchers have reached.

Just as they did in the days of Dr Semmelweis. Ignaz Philipp Semmelweis was a nineteenth century Hungarian physician who proposed that doctors should wash their hands. That doesn't seem completely unreasonable, but his colleagues were not pleased. What possible difference could hand washing make? It was witchcraft, not science. Dr Semmelweis delivered babies in Vienna's main hospital and noticed that childbed fever, which killed a lot of women, was more common in doctor deliveries than midwife ones. Perhaps, he reasoned, it had something to do with doctors delivering babies after doing autopsies. But nobody knew about germs, and the idea that illness could be passed from hand to hand was ridiculed. Semmelweis even improved the mortality rate by making those under his command wash their hands in lime, but the old guard was unimpressed. He died at age 47 in a mental asylum, and was only vindicated years after his death when Louis Pasteur linked disease with bacteria.

Dr Semmelweis has not just bequeathed us an injunction to observe personal hygiene. His story shows how unscientific scientific attitudes can be. In fact, it often takes a very long time for an enquiry to resolve itself into clear lines that everyone can agree on, but decisions still have to be taken. Wait for clear proof and you could wait a lifetime. Instinct and extrapolation have their place.

The people who assert their scientific ethos most emphatically are often those who fail to realise that truth emerges slowly and imperfectly, and that knowledge may evolve decades before certainty. Demanding high-grade proof is just as unscientific as magic crystals. Arguably it is even worse when the demand comes from people who claim to be scientifically unimpeachable.

There is also a lesson from drug testing. Drug companies have to research a new agent for years before the authorities will let them sell it, and we all nod sagely that this is wise. We like high standards when it comes to dangerous things. Except drugs are not just dangerous— they are also helpful. It causes harm to release a drug with toxic side effects, but it also causes harm to withhold a drug that could have saved lives. The higher the bar is set, the safer and more efficacious licensed drugs will be but, concomitantly, more patients will die of things that never got out of the test tube. As any economist will tell you, maximum benefit is a balance between reward and cost. Society must accept risk and uncertainty to get drugs that work.

If we demand functional foods and nutraceuticals prove their worth to an impeccable standard, we lose the good they might have done us. These pages lay out in summary form the evidence that certain key foods and nutraceuticals may promote health by, in particular, suppressing inflammation. There is too much data for informed people to say there is nothing in it, but the picture is not complete. There are many animal experiments that show benefit, some of which are dramatic, but there is always a question mark about how this translates to humans. This is particularly true when the experiment used higher levels of the substance than anyone could eat. There are also experiments that measure the properties of test substances on cell cultures in laboratory dishes. There are population studies, but they invoke a lot of variables. There are detailed observations of the chemistry at a molecular level, which imply efficacy, but cannot prove it.

So the question requires a mind shift. Do not seek certainty. Do not write me a letter quoting your PhD and telling me all the ways I am wrong. The issue is not what is proven, but what is probable and useful.

No one can tell you functional foods and nutraceuticals are a proven good idea, and no one can tell you they are rubbish. There are strong implications, but there is not yet any consensus. Look to professional advisers and you can find any opinion you like, but the point is not to rest everything on what a professional advisor says. What stares you in the face is personal philosophy. You can stick to establishment-grade evidence and be wrong, or right; you can follow your nose, do what seems to be reasonable and likely to work, and be wrong or right as well. You choose.

It is well known that health and long life have a lot to do with eating the right things, mainly coloured plants. It is also well recognised that a large part of the phenomenon comes down to certain elements in those plants, particularly polyphenols (see <u>Nutraceuticals and where they come from</u>). It is a short step in logic to propose that, within reason, health and longevity can be promoted by consuming more of the health-giving parts than a regular diet delivers, and consuming them from novel sources (the range is a critical factor). And if this logic impresses you, you might err on the side of precaution by taking them.

Don't ask professionals what to do. Rely on them for the evidence, which includes new thinking, and a range of informed opinions, and then sort yourself out. You would be mad to take grape seeds for pneumonia but, where the science is still developing, the field of legitimate responses is broad. There is a balance between evidence and experimentation, certainty and possibility, and it is yours to find.

Probably the biggest question is the downside. If the benefit is not pinned down, what is the cost? This is where functional foods have an edge, why health researchers and drug developers are paying them attention, and why they deserve to be part of the health-conscious person's armamentarium. Unless you get seriously silly about it – like carrots for every meal – healthy food will not harm you.[2]

Most drugs carry risks, and people take them because the odds are worth it. The calculation is absent with food – subject, of course, to the discussion that follows in the next chapter about which functional foods and nutraceuticals you should consider. I am not suggesting you consume every supplement in sight.

Often official voices assert that a sensible diet is enough for good health, and extras are superfluous. This is a good point, widely adopted by conservative thinkers, but reasoning beyond it is a key part of the functional food philosophy. The answer is that a traditional diet is enough for average results, but the imperative is to improve on the average. The goal is maximum health, not adequate health. Functional food does not treat a deficiency, it achieves a potential. It is the difference between petrol and rocket fuel.

---

2 An excess of carrots even has a medical name – carotinaemia – and turns the afflicted person yellow, like jaundice. Several cases were reported in Britain during World War II, when normal diets were disrupted. Almond, S., & Logan, R. F. L. (1942). Carotenaemia. *British Medical Journal*, 2(4260), 239–241.

References

Ahmed, F. (2010). Health: Edible advice. *Nature,* 468(7327), S10-S12.

Almond, S, Logan, R.F.L (1942). Carotinaemia. *British Medical Journal,* 2(4260), 239-241.

Best, M., & Neuhauser, D. (2004). Ignaz Semmelweis and the birth of infection control. *Quality & Safety in Health Care,* 13, 233-234.

Bøhn, S., Ward, N., Hodgson, J., & Croft, K. (2012). Effects of tea and coffee on cardiovascular disease risk. *Food & Function,* 3(6), 575-591.

Brandt, K., Christensen, L., Hansen-Møller, J., Hansen, S., Haraldsdottir, J., Jespersen, L., Purup, S., Kharazmi, A., Barkholt, V., Frøkiær, H., & Kobæk-Larsen, M. (2004). Health promoting compounds in vegetables and fruits. *Trends in Food Science & Technology,* 15(7), 384-393.

Carter, B.R. (2004). Childbed Fever: A Scientific Biography of Ignaz Semmelweis. Transaction Publishers.

Mithen, F.R.A.T.H.M. (2011). Challenges in Assessing Health-Promoting Properties of Phytochemicals. *Plant Science and Human Nutrition,* 23(7), 2483.

Moyer, M. (2014). Nutrition: Vitamins on trial. *Nature,* 510(7506), 462-464.

Rajendran, P., Nandakumar, N., Rengarajan, T., Palaniswami, R., Gnanadhas, E., Lakshminarasaiah, U., Gopas, J., & Nishigaki, I. (2014). Antioxidants and human diseases. *Clinica Chimica Acta,* 436, 332-347.

10

BIOAVAILABILITY; GETTING PAST THE BORDER GUARDS

The paradox of hostility to nature's gifts

Whether nutraceuticals really work is controversial, as discussed in Proof of the pudding. A key argument of their detractors, something of a trump card, is the problem of *bioavailability*. Bioavailability refers to the hurdles your diet has to clear before nutrients get to your organs. It has been observed time and again that only tiny amounts of nutraceutical substances get from plate to bloodstream. Turmeric, for instance, is the queen of nutraceuticals, yet when it is eaten, very little turns up in blood samples. Repeatedly nutraceuticals have shown benefits in artificial situations, like a cell culture dish or a chemical reaction – discussed extensively in pages to come – but their promise obviously hinges on getting inside your metabolism. The possibility they might not needs an answer.

In order to simplify something that is not simple there are two hurdles. Firstly, anything you eat must get across the gut wall and, secondly, it must get past your liver. Multiple factors impact on each step, like the way food is prepared or which bowel bugs you carry, but those are the two main issues. Your liver breaks up and eliminates toxins, and it receives the blood from your gut before the general circulation does in case you eat something nasty. So your diet has to get through the gut wall's elaborate filtering system and past the gauntlet of enzymes in the liver before it turns up in your bloodstream and starts the journey to organs that need it.

Even essential things can have limited bioavailability, but this does not spell the death knell for their nutritional usefulness. Iron, for instance, is vital, and present in a lot of different foods, yet many people are deficient because only one short piece of the human bowel can absorb it.

Bioavailability is the reason fibre is a laxative – it passes straight through – and one of the reasons some drugs are injected (that is, straight into blood, never mind the hurdles). Limits on bioavailability are rather useful. You don't want every nasty thing you eat getting through security, particularly if you lived in the era before food came clean and wrapped. However, like many of nature's good ideas, there can be overkill. Useful things get tossed out with the bad ones.

It may at first seem strange that phytochemicals, widely touted as keeping us well as we age, struggle to clear the hurdles. However, it meshes with the hormesis theory, previously discussed, that many longevity-promoting polyphenols are mildly toxic. They developed to repel browsers, particularly insects, but they are paradoxes: although the plant's intention was hostile, its phytochemicals keep us well by gently and consistently stimulating our cell-repair machinery. But our metabolisms have noticed the toxicity, so nature has tilted the available defences towards keeping them out. Conventional drugs get the same treatment, which is why most drugs are taken several times a day. However, low bioavailability is not the end of the question.

For a start, measuring what gets through is not straightforward, particularly with single doses or the short time periods used in a laboratory. The blood-borne consequence of one serving of the key food may be too small or the tests too non-specific to capture what is going on. The molecules of interest may not be easy to find in a blood sample, and few studies have ever gone beyond blood samples and tried to measure them inside tissues or cells.

And the molecule of interest might not even be known. Polyphenols break up into smaller molecules when they are digested and absorbed and their therapeutic effects may well be driven by their fragments. The chemistry of biological molecules is astonishingly complex, and a challenge to unravel, even in the modern era. The degradation of the curcumin in turmeric, for instance, has been well studied yet papers continue to debate its details. For other nutraceuticals the picture is even more obscure. Just what is impacting where can't be stated with any certainty.

There is also evidence polyphenols may not rely on detectable concentrations to work. Certain elegant experiments show they can deliver key longevity functions, on cell signals and gene reading, at vanishingly small levels. Drugs are routinely detected in blood samples, and perhaps the establishment expects from this example that all metabolically active molecules can be detected similarly. Perhaps drugs are not a useful comparison for the subtlety of low-key natural options.

Polyphenols can also accumulate. Even if the amounts getting through are tiny, they can lodge over time in their targets. This is a vital consideration for effects that take years to play out. One study fed pigs on blueberries, and chased the polyphenol anthocyanins – the blue part of blueberries – through their systems.[1] Although none were found in their blood, they turned up later in autopsies of their liver and brains. Likewise, rats were fed blackberries and 12 days later, anthocyanins were found in various organs, including their hearts.[2]

---

1 Fernandes, I., Faria, A., Freitas, V., Calhau, C., & Mateus, N. (2015). Multiple-approach studies to assess anthocyanin bioavailability. *Phytochemistry Reviews*, 14(6), 899-919.
2 Fernandes, I., Faria, A., Freitas, V., Calhau, C., & Mateus, N. (2015). Multiple-approach studies to assess anthocyanin bioavailability. Phytochemistry Reviews, 14(6), 899-919.

Anthocyanins are some of the least bioavailable polyphenols, yet berries red, blue and black, in which they feature, and purple plants generally, are some of the healthiest on offer. Accumulation may well be the explanation. Accumulation has also been shown with epicatechin, the major polyphenol in chocolate.

And maybe getting out of the gut is not a problem, because the gut is enough. As discussed in The secret garden, robust and diverse species of bowel bacteria are key to maintaining a healthy bowel wall which stops inflammation-inducing molecules slipping through. A variety of major nutraceuticals including curcumin (from turmeric), catechin (from tea), and grape seeds seem to help. Bowel bacteria are exquisitely sensitive to what you eat, because it is the same as what they eat, and tentative evidence implies plant polyphenols are a useful part of the mix.

So blood samples are not the end of the issue. There is far more to the complexity of natural anti-inflammatories than whether a standard lab assay can find them.

References

Aggarwal, B.B., Gupta, S.C., & Sung, B. (2018). Curcumin: an orally bioavailable blocker of TNF and other pro-inflammatory biomarkers. *British Journal of Pharmacology,* 169(8), 1672-1692.

Bohn, T., Gordon, McDougall, J., Alegría, A., Alminger, M., Arrigoni, E., Aura, A., Brito, C., Cilla, A., El, S.N., Karakaya, S., Martínez-Cuesta, M.C., & Santos, C.N. (2015). "Mind the gap—deficits in our knowledge of aspects impacting the bioavailability of phytochemicals and their metabolites—a position paper focusing on carotenoids and polyphenols." *Molecular Nutrition & Food Research,* 59(7), 1307-1323.

D'Archivio, M., Filesi, C., Rosaria, V., Scazzocchio, B., & Masella, R. (2010). Bioavailability of the Polyphenols: Status and Controversies. *International Journal of Molecular Sciences,* 11(4), 1321-1342.

Del Rio, D., Rodriguez-Mateos, A., Spencer, J., Tognolini, M., Borges, G., & Crozier, A. (2013). *Antioxidants & Redox Signaling,* 18(14), 1818-1892.

Edwards, C., Havlik, J., Cong, W., Mullen, W., Preston, T., Morrison, D., & Combet, E. (2017). Polyphenols and health: Interactions between fibre, plant polyphenols and the gut microbiota. *Nutrition Bulletin,* 42(4), 356-360.

Fernandes, I., Faria, A., Freitas, V., Calhau, C., & Mateus, N. (2015). Multiple-approach studies to assess anthocyanin bioavailability. *Phytochemistry Reviews,* 14(6), 899-919.

Figueira, I., Menezes, R., Macedo, D., Costa, I., & Nunes dos Santos, C. (2017). Polyphenols Beyond Barriers: A Glimpse into the Brain. *Current Neuropharmacology,* 15(4), 562-594.

Ho, C., SiuWai, C., Fung, M., & Benzie, I. (2017). Tea polyphenols: absorption, bioavailability and potential toxicity. *CAB Reviews,* 12(2), 1-22.

Lopresti, A. (2018). The Problem of Curcumin and Its Bioavailability: Could Its Gastrointestinal Influence Contribute to Its Overall Health-Enhancing Effects? *Advances in Nutrition,* 9(1), 41-50.

Pressman, P., Clemens, R., & Hayes, A. (2017). Bioavailability of micronutrients obtained from supplements and food. *Toxicology Research and Application,* 1, 1.

Russo, G., Tedesco, I., Spagnuolo, C., & Russo, M. (2017). Antioxidant polyphenols in cancer treatment: Friend, foe or foil? *Seminars in Cancer Biology,* 46, 1-13.

Scheepens, A., Tan, K., & Paxton, J.W. (2010). Improving the oral bioavailability of beneficial polyphenols through designed synergies. *Genes & Nutrition,* 5(1), 75-87.

Schneider, C., Gordon, O.N., Edwards, R.L., & Luis, P.B. (2015). Degradation of curcumin: From mechanism to biological implications. *Journal of Agricultural and Food Chemistry,* 63(35), 7606-7614.

Selma, M.V., Espín, J.C., Tomás-Barberán, F.A.(2009). Interaction between phenolics and gut microbiota: role in human health. *Journal of Agricultural and Food Chemistry,* 57(15), 6485-501.

Tresserra-Rimbau, A., Lamuela-Raventos, R.M., Moreno, J.J. (2018). Polyphenols, food and pharma. Current knowledge and directions for future research. *Biochemical Pharmacology,* 156, 186-195.

Yang, C., Sang, S., Lambert, J., & Lee, M. (2008). Bioavailability issues in studying the health effects of plant polyphenolic compounds. *Molecular Nutrition & Food Research,* 52(S1), S139-S151.

11

ORTHOREXIA NERVOSA;
THE WRONG WAY TO EAT RIGHT
Evangelical eating and how to avoid it

For decades wellness-conscious people have embraced vegetables, rejected sugar and observed all the other well-established choices that create a good diet. This book, as you will know if you got this far, argues that the next step is food with functionality. For balance, it is necessary to cite the key pitfall. Doctors call it *orthorexia nervosa* (*ortho* means 'straight' or 'upright' as in orthodox), and everyone else calls it 'taking it too far.' The search for ultimate nutrition does not mean sausages are poisonous or that nothing should be cooked, but unfortunately, food rules can get out of hand.

The term orthorexia nervosa was coined in 1997 by a doctor called Steven Bratman who wrote about his own experience.[1] Dr Bratman developed his diet to the point that he wouldn't eat vegetables picked more than 15 minutes earlier, and he chewed every mouthful 50 times. After coming to his senses, he realised he had found a new condition. He defined it as 'a fixation on eating proper food.'

The term orthorexia nervosa does not appear in any official classification of mental illness. It is an informal description and, as with all new ideas, there is academic debate about what it is and where

---

1   Bratman, S. (1997). Health Food Junkie. *Yoga Journal*, 42-50.

its parameters lie. It has certain things in common with other eating problems, like anorexia nervosa, although it is not about weight; orthorexia nervosa sufferers are happy to eat, but fixate on quality. It also overlaps with obsessive-compulsive disorders where people wash their hands too often and touch every lamp post as they walk down the street.

People with orthorexia nervosa believe the right food is pure and must not be contaminated, even with other food. It must be rigidly seasonal, or uniformly raw, or macrobiotic (food with yin and yang in balance), or uncut (to preserve the energy field), or washed (to remove contaminants) or unwashed (to retain nutrients). It must be what cavemen ate, it must be right for your blood type, it must be right for the time of day. Sugar is poisonous, or meat is, or milk, or 'deadly nightshade' (potatoes and tomatoes), or onions or bread. Knives and pots cannot be used if they touched the wrong food, even when they have been washed.

This is fanaticism. Some of the rules, like avoiding meat or sugar, are valid choices. The issue is how vigorously they are pursued. A balanced person does not recoil in alarm from a jelly bean. Other rules are absurd and scientifically baseless.

Affected people start well, but become fixated over time on certain choices and complex principles. They spend hours researching and hunting down the 'right' options. The Internet, as with everything, accelerates the journey of anyone who goes looking. There are websites and blogs for every silly idea, and no shortage of encouragement for the novice. The issue takes on the aura of a religious or philosophical crusade; there is one true way, and everything must be sacrificed to follow it. Understandably, a feature of the condition is a strained social life.

People who go down this path might even feel better for it. Adopting a new philosophy creates a positive vibe, which makes a person see their health in a new and rosier light. The mind plays such tricks, and the consequences are powerful. For instance, a new drug must always be tested – the law demands it – on people who do not know whether they are getting the real thing or a sugar pill. This is because merely taking a pill by itself convinces users they feel better. So it is with food philosophies. Proponents feel healthier because they expect to. The time and energy they spend finding and cooking (or, in the case of raw food variants, not cooking) exotic food options adds to the impression.

The reality is different. People on extreme diets often have deficiencies of essential micronutrients like vitamins, and lose unhealthy levels of weight. They spend inordinate time and money on their obsession. They feel anxious about observing all the rules, and experience guilt about eating a tiny amount of the wrong thing. Food gets stripped of comfort, sociability and, ironically, the principles of good health that really matter.

A short step in logic takes the problem into the world of supplements. If certain supplements are a good idea, a few more would be even better. When you have a shopping bag full of pill bottles you have lost the plot. Unfortunately, it is not difficult to do. There are hundreds of options for people who want a little extra zing in a tablet, all of which come with their own justifications ranging from the credible to the bizarre. A raft of literature has been written to promote them to the buying public and explain the theories behind them. Discovering new and exciting supplements provides hours of stimulation for a dedicated health junkie. It appeals to the collecting urge, the researching urge and the urge to exert control. There also seems to be a theme, popular among health zealots, that anything that did not originate from the medical establishment is 'natural' and therefore desirable.

Few countries regulate supplements with any vigour, and the marriage of soft science with commerce turns over billions worldwide. The biggest imperative for the wise is knowing how to navigate the options.

And that is the problem with advocating a new way of looking at diet, and why this point is a chapter in the book. I do not want to give succour to any cults of evangelical eating. Supplements and food with bioactive anti-inflammatories are likely to do you good, in my view, but the benefits do not multiply without limit. Twenty supplements a day are not twenty times better than one. And supplements do not replace whole food, nor does all whole food have to be the most nutritionally dense possible. Supplements are called supplements because they are add-ons, not the main course.

References

Bratman, S., & Dunn, T. (2016). On orthorexia nervosa: A review of the literature and proposed diagnostic criteria. *Eating Behaviors.*

Bratman, S. (1997). Health Food Junkie. *Yoga Journal,* 42-50.

Bratman, S. & Knight, D. (2000). Health Food Junkies. Overcoming the Obsession with Healthful eating. *Broadway Books.*

Missbach, B., Hinterbuchinger, B., Dreiseitl, V., Zellhofer, S., Kurz, C., & König, J. (2015). When Eating Right, Is Measured Wrong! A Validation and Critical Examination of the ORTO-15 Questionnaire in German. *PLoS ONE,* 10(8), e0135772.

Brytek-Matera, A., Donini, L., Krupa, M., Poggiogalle, E., & Hay, P. (2015). Orthorexia nervosa and self-attitudinal aspects of body image in female and male university students. *Journal of Eating Disorders,* 3.

Brytek-Matera, A., Fonte, M., Poggiogalle, E., Donini, L., & Cena, H. (2017). Orthorexia nervosa: relationship with obsessive-compulsive symptoms, disordered eating patterns and body uneasiness among Italian university students. *Eating and Weight Disorders—Studies on Anorexia, Bulimia and Obesity,* 22(4), 609-617.

12

SPOILED FOR CHOICE

How to navigate the functional food smorgasbord

If you are convinced – or at least intrigued – the obvious question is which supplements or functional foods to add to your diet. There is no shortage of people open to the idea. It is estimated up to seventy per cent of Americans take some sort of supplement and presumably a fair few elsewhere follow them.[1] The industry is worth multiple billions. Unfortunately, pointing to what works involves another spin on the implications versus evidence carousel, but nonetheless, guiding principles can be elucidated.

First, mind the flotsam (and there is a lot of it). There is money to be made selling boiled beetle juice and tincture of geranium to the worried well and the fashion-conscious tonic imbiber. Many companies do, but I am not going to give examples as I do not want lawyers' letters. There are rules of thumb for spotting the industry's excess baggage, particularly the headlines. Ignore products that cite the diets of romanticised eras like the Incas. Likewise, ignore those that emphasise exotic sources like rainforests and alpine meadows. Pass over ones that refer to vagaries like energy boosting. Pay no attention to puff like 'natural'—tobacco is natural too, as is radiation

1   Ronis, M.J.J., Pedersen, K.B., & Watt, J. (2017). Adverse Effects of Nutraceuticals and Dietary Supplements. Annu Rev Pharmacol Toxicol.

(the sun makes it). Above all else, when the product is touted for healing major diseases, particularly the incurable kind, leave the shop walking backwards.[2]

Do not be seduced by single ingredient additives, because there aren't many that work. Iodine and folic acid do, and are added to the food supply for sound biological reasons. Vitamin D is useful for the frail elderly, and possibly others; the science is evolving. People who eat too much processed food might have mild vitamin deficiencies and benefit from supplemental ones, but the experts debate that. No matter – it is unlikely the cheese burger brigade will seek guidance from this book. Otherwise vitamins and essential elements, in pills not food, work for people with medically diagnosed deficiencies but not for anyone else. Your metabolism only needs tiny amounts of micronutrients for good health which a balanced diet delivers, and more is not better.

Useful substances, like anti-inflammatories, function best with the many other molecules that nature created them to coexist with. Isolating a single useful molecule (or the one that appears to be useful), and cooking it up in a tank doesn't necessarily work. This vital point was discussed more fully in The orchestra, not the soloist.

Whole food which has been tweaked is also something to approach with caution. Plant sterols added to food like margarine appear to reduce cholesterol, although official voices remain wary of them. Milk that lacks the A1 protein may have some anti-inflammatory potential but the evidence is still being gathered. It also matters whether the base food is healthy. Hamburgers that combine oats with red meat may be better for you, but that does not mean you should eat more of them.

---

2   There is work underway to determine if some nutraceuticals, such as ginger (for nausea) and green tea, might have a role in treating cancer and its symptoms. This is highly experimental and requires medical supervision.

Sometimes the silliness is obvious. Water with added oxygen is nonsense (to get more oxygen open your mouth), as is collagen in beer (to make your skin glow while you get drunk!) and numerous other excesses of the industrial food world.

There is some evidence for targeted supplements like St John's wort for depression and red yeast rice for high cholesterol, but they are treatments for disease, and are therefore outside the scope of this book. There is also a lot of room to be sceptical about treatments touted for common and difficult problems like body weight and fatigue. The commercial incentives behind them are considerable, given the number of people who want a solution, and personal medical advice is obligatory.

In the same vein, look carefully at the more unusual offerings. Some herbs labelled 'traditional Chinese' may cause kidney injury; others (black cohosh, red clover) contain compounds similar to oestrogen and may increase breast cancer risk. Consult your doctor if you take prescription drugs as there can be multiple points of interaction, particularly with the risk of bleeding. Pregnancy, known or possible (risk is greatest at the outset), is a serious red flag against taking anything your professional advisor doesn't know about.

Be wary of the mainstream media, at least at the populist end. Significant findings are often reported when major scientific journals publish them, but they usually appear without the underlying controversies. Experts always debate new trial findings, and proper understanding needs a grasp of how well the trial was designed as well as insights from previous trials, laboratory experiments and everything else that bears on the question. Newspaper headlines are written to turn your head. They may or may not represent good advice.

The best starting point is something closely related to whole food or, for something that is not a routine food, like grape seeds, a whole natural product.

It is a lesson drug developers have noticed: modern thinking in the drug-designing world is that shotguns that block multiple pathways are better than snipers that target just one, especially for complex long-term diseases like cancer. Much like food, really.

Whichever options appeal, do your homework. Read up on the ones with the best evidence – the rest of this book is a good start – then commit to them. The benefits take years, so there is no room for dabbling. And don't expect to feel better. A daily dose of natural anti-inflammatories will not deliver energy and glowing skin if you were living sensibly already. The point is to massage cellular signalling cascades and read the right genes to keep vital organs healthy and thereby live longer than you otherwise would, not just to take a tonic.

Above all else, do not rely on functional food to compensate for the rest of your lifestyle. Taking a pill or a powder or a pomegranate smoothie is not an isolated panacea, that will get you into the centenarian's club on its own. The touted benefit is fine tuning a lifestyle that already ticks obvious boxes of reasonable exercise and sensible eating. Longevity still relies in the main on eating a comprehensive array of minimally processed plants; regular muscle and brain activity; and doing what your doctor says re blood pressure, cholesterol, cancer screening and drinking. You will never live your best or your longest on functional food alone.

References

Barbagallo, C.M., Cefalù, A.B., Noto, D., & Averna, M.R. (2015). Role of Nutraceuticals in Hypolipidemic Therapy. *Frontiers in Cardiovascular Medicine*, 11(2).

Birringer, M. (2011). Hormetics: Dietary Triggers of an Adaptive Stress Response. *Pharmaceutical Research*, 28(11), 2680-2694.

Brooke-Taylor, S., Dwyer, K., Woodford, K., & Kost, N. (2017). Systematic Review of the Gastrointestinal Effects of A1 Compared with A2 β-Casein. *Advances in Nutrition*, 8(5), 739-748.

Curel, P. (2013). Studies of supplements highlight harms. *Reactions Weekly*, 1374(1).

Frantz, S. (2005). Drug discovery: Playing dirty *Nature*, 437, 942-943.

Köhler, J., Teupser, D., Elsässer, A., & Weingärtner, O. (2017). Plant sterol enriched functional food and atherosclerosis. *British Journal of Pharmacology*, 174(11), 1281-1289.

Moyer, M. (2014). Nutrition: Vitamins on trial. *Nature*, 510(7506), 462-464.

Poljsak, B., Šuput, D., & Milisav, I. (2011). Review Article Achieving the Balance between ROS and Antioxidants: When to Use the Synthetic Antioxidants. *Oxidative Medicine and Cellular Longevity*.

Ronis, M.J.J., Pedersen, K.B., & Watt, J. (2017). Adverse Effects of Nutraceuticals and Dietary Supplements. *Annual Review of Pharmacology and Toxicology*.

Ulbricht, C., & Chao, W. (2010). Phytochemicals in the Oncology Setting. *Current Treatment Options in Oncology*, 11(3), 95-106.

Weingärtner, O., Baber, R., & Teupser, D. (2014). Plant sterols in food: No consensus in guidelines. *Biochemical and Biophysical Research Communications*, 446(3), 811-813.

DR. RODERICK MULGAN: THE INTERNAL FLAME

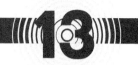

KEEPING THE LINES OPEN

Heart attacks and strokes

Blood is like electricity: cut off the supply and everything downstream dies. A heart attack, which kills a piece of heart, and a stroke, which kills a piece of brain, are both diseases of abrupt obstruction.[1] They occur because the supply lines to hearts and brains are minute: the coronary arteries which feed the heart – hence the term 'coronary' for a heart attack – are thinner than a pencil; the ones in the brain are even tinier. Our two most critical organs depend on dangerously narrow portals, and it doesn't take much to block one.

What we call heart disease is really disease of arteries. In fact everything lives on blood, not just your heart and brain, and critical supply points abound. Obstructed leg arteries make calf muscles ache with walking. The kidneys filter out impurities and struggle when blood they work on can't get through. These things wait for you as you get older and will drag down your quality of life, if you are lucky (because if you aren't lucky, they will kill you).

The state of your blood vessels is vital to staying alive and healthy. If you want to live long, and live well, you need robust ones.

---

1   For the sake of completeness, I state that some strokes reflect blood vessel rupture, not blockage, and that some of the blockages come from floating blood clots, not the atherosclerosis described herein. These events are the minority.

What causes blockages?

So the nub of the issue is the blockages. What are they and where do they come from?

The answer is fat or, more properly, a blip of fat called atherosclerosis. Atherosclerosis is a fatty lump that grows inside an artery wall. We all have them and they take decades to develop. As we go about our lives, and age, they slowly form inside us. In the end, one of them will grow large enough to cause trouble. It will block off an essential conduit, and part of a vital organ will die. Possibly, so may you.

Atherosclerosis is the biggest disease in the First World. More people in the developed part of the planet die of heart attacks than of any other single cause, and many of the rest die of a stroke. More people suffer these diseases without dying. They live for years with shortness of breath and paralysis. And not just men: contrary to public perception, heart disease is also the number one killer of women. The prime menace to humanity is not a plague bacillus, a nuclear warhead or a planet-killing space rock. It is a teaspoon of fat.

Fortunately, you can do something about it. The World Health Organisation estimates that up to ninety per cent of people who die of heart attacks had at least one lifestyle risk factor or, in other words, something they could have changed.[2] This is Framingham's legacy (see Dealing with destiny). The way we live, and the choices we make, determine whether atherosclerotic lumps grow quickly and kill us prematurely, or grow slowly and carry us off at the conclusion of a healthy life lived actively to the end.

It is advice you know well. If you keep your weight down, if you exercise, if you eat more plants and less meat, if you eat fish and don't smoke, your atherosclerotic lumps are likely to grow slowly. If you fill your system with animal fat and lie around so everything gets sluggish,

---

2   Mackay, J., & Mensah, G. (2004). The Atlas of Heart Disease and Stroke. *World Health Organisation.*

you will have dangerous ones by middle age. So until the 1970s, that was that. We knew where we were, we knew what to do. Run your life properly, do what the doctor said (which is the same as what Framingham said) and you were doing all you could. But science does not stay still. The next chapter was just about to open.

The next frontier: Inflammation

Everyone used to think the atherosclerotic lumps of fat were passive, like driftwood at a bend in a river. Eat enough fat and it will stick there. Keep eating fat and the lump will get bigger. One day, you will have yourself a blockage. It all made sense.

Except it is not that simple: since the 1970s a new view has progressively intruded into the consciousness of people who study these things, and pointed to a deeper explanation. The lump is not passive, and it is not a rubbish tip. The lump is alive. The fat doesn't just sit there, it provokes an angry response. It is an intruder that refuses to go away and it stirs up the same response as any other unwelcome guest. The lump is a centre of inflammatory reactions. It is a fizzing seat of chemical processes, a dance of fat molecules and protein cascades and white blood cells. One authority characterises the whole atherosclerosis phenomenon as 'a multifactorial, smouldering, immune-inflammatory disease of… arteries fuelled by lipids.'[3]

The revelation should not have been a shock. Our old nineteenth-century friend Rudolf Virchow looked at fatty artery deposits down a microscope and noticed white blood cells in them. The implication seemed pretty obvious: 'In some, particularly violent cases the softening manifests itself even in the arteries not as the consequence of a really fatty process, but as a direct product of inflammation.'[4]

---

3   Falk, E. (2006). Pathogenesis of atherosclerosis. *Journal of the American College of Cardiology,* 47(8).
4   Libby, P. (2012). History of Discovery: Inflammation in Atherosclerosis. *Arteriosclerosis, Thrombosis, and Vascular Biology,* 32, 2045-2051.

Yet his insight died with him. His words were there for anyone to read (and read them they did for he is a widely studied figure), and the same evidence – white cells in the atherosclerosis – were seen by everyone who looked down a microscope at artery walls. It didn't matter. For over a hundred years there was no groundswell of excitement about the explanatory power of inflammation. Fat got stuck and that was that. In the last four decades, Virchow's view has been revived, to the point where few dispute it, and it points to a much better understanding of what is going on.

It starts with cholesterol, the world's most notorious fat molecule. The Framingham research had stated it was a problem, and numerous other studies had agreed, so authorities have been shouting themselves hoarse telling everyone to lay off it. Except laying off it is not straightforward. You consume it if you eat meat, milk or eggs – which most people do – but you also make your own in your liver. You can't eliminate it – even vegans can't – nor would you want to as it is very useful. The walls of all your cells are made of it. Without cholesterol there would be no you. The problem is cholesterol's dark side: notwithstanding its indispensability, cholesterol is a hazard.

Cholesterol starts from your gut (what you eat) and your liver (what you make) and travels via the blood without incident. Our defence system recognises normal molecules and leaves them alone, otherwise we would be dead from friendly fire. But when cholesterol lodges in an artery wall it forms a bond with oxygen atoms. That makes it a different molecule. The call goes out that an intruder has been detected. Your body thinks it is a wooden splinter and calls in the blood cells of inflammation. That is what Virchow was seeing when he looked at slides cut from arteries.

Despite the popular obsession with cholesterol, one half of heart attacks and strokes happen in people with normal levels, and people with the same level differ widely in their incidence of blood vessel disease.[5] Mice that lack genes for key inflammatory proteins have a greatly curtailed incidence of atherosclerotic deposits, regardless of their cholesterol.[6] So cholesterol, despite its notoriety, is not the full story. The issue is what goes with it.

In the early stages, white blood cells wrap themselves around the oxidised cholesterol. Pathologists call them *foam cells* because masses under the microscope look like surf. They form a *fatty streak*, a line of fat-filled cells like streaky bacon. Over decades, the lesion becomes a bump, which sticks out and disrupts blood flow. By age 50, eighty-five per cent of people will have significant atherosclerosis, even though they feel healthy.[7] Eventually some of these lesions will cause a partial obstruction. Angina, for instance, is heart pain on exercise, and it happens because partially obstructed arteries let enough blood through for resting but not enough for exertion. *Claudication* is the name for the same thing in leg muscles. All most undesirable, but not the real problem. The real problem is a lesion that bursts; a burst bubble is the most dangerous of all.

As a bump gets old, the cells in its centre die and release their cholesterol. They turn into soft-centre chocolates, runny in the middle. That is where the name comes from: "athero" means a porridge like gruel, and "sclerosis" means hardening. Atherosclerosis is a rigid scar with porridge in the middle. Eventually the inflammatory cells wear the cap away completely and disaster ensues.

The disaster is the meeting between porridge and blood. It is not a happy one, because blood is cued for self-preservation. Nicks and cuts are part of going about in the world, so when blood detects anything

5   Wick, G., & Grundtman, C. (eds). (2012). Inflammation and atherosclerosis. *Springer-Verlay/Wien*.
6   Falk, E. (2006). Pathogenesis of atherosclerosis. *Journal of the American College of Cardiology*, 47(8).
7   Weintraub, H. (2008). Identifying the vulnerable patient with rupture-prone plaque. *American Journal of Cardiology*, 101(supple) ,3F-10F.

unusual, floating proteins clump together to form a clot. That is why you don't bleed forever when you cut yourself. The downside is that blood may clot even when it is the last thing you want, such as when the corridor is running with porridge. The porridge calls down the clumping reaction and closes the channel. That is why heart attacks and strokes are so abrupt (the name 'stroke' refers to instant paralysis). You walk around for decades with atherosclerosis in your heart or brain, then one day it ruptures and releases the porridge. A clot forms and cuts off the blood flow: instant chest pain, instant incapacity.

Beyond the microscope

Virchow started it by looking down a microscope, but multiple lines of modern evidence go beyond what can be seen and keep turning up the same message.

Inflammation releases protein markers and white blood cells into the bloodstream which doctors routinely measure and make deductions from. Comparing them with heart disease is not straightforward, but numerous studies show levels correlate with heart attack risk.[8] Where patients already have a heart issue, such as chest pain, elevated markers mean a higher risk of a worse outcome.

Inflammation also provides a deeper explanation for cardiac pharmaceuticals. By the 1960s, most researchers said cholesterol was bad for you, but people like eating fat, so the hunt started for a cholesterol-busting drug. Most candidates were uninspired, until the late 1980s when statins arrived. The simple concept of blocking the enzyme that makes cholesterol has made them the most widely prescribed class of drugs in the world. Undoubtedly, statins work. Large population studies show they reduce heart attacks by anything

---

8   Libby, P., Ridker, P., & Hansson G. (2009). Inflammation in artherosclerosis. From pathophysiology to practice. *Journal of the American College of Cardiology,* 54(23).

from twenty-five to forty-five per cent.[9] Over 200 million people take one every day, and they are so effective some doctors recommend they should be automatically offered to everyone over fifty.[10]

But there appears to be more to it than reducing cholesterol. Inflammatory blood markers are reduced by statins, independent of any effect on cholesterol. Just as heart attacks happen in plenty of people with normal cholesterol, statins reduce hearts attacks in people with normal cholesterol as well. People with elevated blood markers for inflammation but low cholesterol benefit from statins, but people with low cholesterol and low inflammatory markers do not.[11] It implies there is more to it than reducing cholesterol, and one of the prime explanations is the ability of statins to suppress inflammation.

Statins inhibit NF-κB, reduce levels of cytokines and inhibit the ingress of white cells (see Inflammation, nuts and bolts). Just how much of the benefit comes from reducing cholesterol, and how much from blocking inflammation, remains to be clarified, but no one doubts these wildly successful drugs are inflammation-busters on multiple fronts.

Another early Framingham insight was the effect of high blood pressure, often called hypertension. We need some pressure in our vessels to move the blood along, but too much is damaging because it wears the vessel lining and provides cholesterol with a way in. Doctors have drugs that lower it, and a major activity of modern doctors, particularly community ones, is measuring blood pressure and finding people who need treatment.

---

9   Jukema, J., Cannon, C., de Craen, A, et al. (2012). The Controversies of Statin Therapy. *Journal of the American Journal of Cardiology*, 60(10), 875-881.

10 Grundy, S.M. (2014). Statins for All? *The American Journal of Cardiology*, 114(9), 1443-1446.

11 Antonopoulos, A.S., Margaritis, M., Lee, R,, Channon, K., & Antoniades, C. (2012). Statins as Anti-Inflammatory Agents in Atherogenesis: Molecular Mechanisms and Lessons from the Recent Clinical Trials. *Current Pharmaceutical Design*, 18(11), 1519-1530.

Blood pressure is the sum of factors like heart rate and the diameter of the tubes the blood is pushed down, and these factors are controlled by nerves and hormones. There is a lot of debate about how it all fits together, but intriguing clues are emerging that inflammation is not far away. Inflammatory cytokines from peripheral tissues leak from the blood into the brain at the very points that control blood pressure. Inflammatory blood markers rise when hypertension is present – and may even rise before blood pressure does – and predict the people who will become hypertensive down the track.[12] Mice that lack inflammatory white cells do not get hypertension when they eat salt, or take hormones that usually raise blood pressure, but they do when white cells are restored.[13]

One key hormone, called *angiotension II*, is made by the kidneys, and has various effects on blood pressure such as making artery muscles constrict. Many consider it the most important mediator of all, and recent work has shown it has multiple pro-inflammatory effects including in the pressure-control regions of the brain. There are blood pressure drugs which stop angiotension II forming and they have a sterling record of reducing heart attacks. But there seems to be more to them than just bringing down blood pressure. They also block some inflammation pathways and this appears to explain at least some of their benefit on blood vessel health.

In fact various hypertension drugs, which prevent heart disease in clinical trials, have been shown to antagonise parts of the inflammation pathway. It has long been accepted that they are effective because they lower blood pressure. It is now apparent there is more to it, and

---

12 Pickering, T. (2007). Stress, Inflammation and Hypertension. *Journal of Clinical Hypertension*, 9 (7).
13 Marvar, P., Lob, H., Vinh, A., Zarreen, F., & Harrison, D. (2011). The central nervous system and inflammation in hypertension. *Current Opinion in Pharmacology*, 11(2), 156-161.

that maybe at least part of their ability to extend life is their anti-inflammatory effect.

The future

Where is all this heading? The next generation of heart drugs are likely to be novel inflammation-blockers, and some very innovative ideas are being tested.

Certain steroids are powerful anti-inflammatories, but they poison almost every organ and are used sparingly. One of the brightest ideas out of the starting blocks comes from nanotechnology and proposes that steroids be delivered directly to the atherosclerotic plaque in a tiny bubble wrapped in a membrane. Trials of this concept are underway.

Another idea is to turn the inflammatory artillery in a useful direction. Vaccination alerts the immune system to notice certain molecules, such as those on a virus, and clear them away if they appear. If people could be vaccinated against oxidised cholesterol, so the theory goes, the inflammatory system would clear it away before it gets stuck somewhere and starts causing trouble. One day a jab against heart disease may be as common as the annual flu shot.

Regardless, inflammation is the foundation of what goes wrong with our blood vessels as we age, and longevity is an exercise in all the measures we can apply that suppress it.

References

Antonopoulos, A.S., Margaritis, M., Lee, R, Channon, K., & Antoniades, C. (2012). Statins as Anti-Inflammatory Agents in Atherogenesis: Molecular Mechanisms and Lessons from the Recent Clinical Trials. *Current Pharmaceutical Design*, 18(11), 1519-1530.

Blaha, M.J., & Martin, S.S (2013). How Do Statins Work? *Journal of the American College of Cardiology*, 62(25), 2392-2394.

Cheryl, L., & Fernando, E. (2010). Inflammation and Therapy for Hypertension. *Current Hypertension Reports*, 12(4), 233-242.

Douglas, P.S., Fiolkoski, J., Berko, B., & Reichek, N. (1988). Echocardiographic visualization of coronary artery anatomy in the adult. *Journal of the American College of Cardiology*, 11(3), 565-571.

Falk, E. (2006). Pathogenesis of atherosclerosis. *Journal of the American College of Cardiology*, 47(8).

Grundy, S.M. (2014). Statins for All? *The American Journal of Cardiology*, 114(9), 1443-1446.

Ikonomidis, I., Michalakeas, C.A., Parissis, J., Paraskevaidis, I., Ntai, K., Papadakis, I., Anastasiou-Nana, M., & Lekakis, J. (2012). Inflammatory markers in coronary artery disease. *BioFactors, (Electronic)*, 38(5), 320-328.

Jukema, J., Cannon, C., de Craen, A, et al. (2012). The Controversies of Statin Therapy. *The American Journal of Cardiology*, 60(10), 875-881.

Kang, J., Toma, I., Sipos, A., McCulloch, F., & Peti-Peterdi, J. (2006). Imaging the renin–angiotensin system: An important target of anti-hypertensive therapy. *Advanced Drug Delivery Reviews*, 58(7), 824-833.

Kinlay, S., & Selwyn, A.P. (2003). Effects of statins on inflammation in patients with acute and chronic coronary syndromes. *The American Journal of Cardiology*, 91(4), 9-13.

Libby, P. (2012). History of Discovery: Inflammation in Atherosclerosis. *Arteriosclerosis, Thrombosis, and Vascular Biology*, 32, 2045-2051.

Libby, P., Ridker, P., & Hansson G. (2009). Inflammation in artherosclerosis. From pathophysiology to practice. *Journal of the American College of Cardiology*, 54(23).

Mackay, J., & Mensah, G. (2004). The Atlas of Heart Disease and Stroke. *World Health Organisation*.

Mahesh, P., & Michael, B. (2013). Inflammation and Atherosclerosis: Disease Modulating Therapies. *Current Treatment Options in Cardiovascular Medicine*, 15(6), 681-695.

Marvar, P., Lob, H., Vinh, A., Zarreen, F., & Harrison, D. (2011). The central nervous system and inflammation in hypertension. *Current Opinion in Pharmacology*, 11(2), 156-161.

Matsuura, E., Hughes, G., & Khamashta, M. (2008). Oxidation of LDL and its clinical implication. *Autoimmunity Reviews*, 7(7), 558-566.

Montecucco, F., & Mach, F. (2009). Statins, ACE inhibitors and ARBs in cardiovascular disease. *Best Practice & Research Clinical Endocrinology & Metabolism*, 23(3), 389-400.

Nilsson, J., Lichtman, A., & Tedgui, A. (2015). Atheroprotective immunity and cardiovascular disease: therapeutic opportunities and challenges. *Journal of Internal Medicine*, 278(5), 507-519.

Paolo, C., Golia, E., & Yeh, E. (2009). CRP and the risk of atherosclerotic events. *Seminars in Immunopathology*, 31(1), 79-94.

Pickering, T. (2007). Stress, Inflammation, and Hypertension. *Journal of Clinical Hypertension,* 9(7).

Shah, P., Chyu, K., Dimayuga, P., & Nilsson, J. (2014). Vaccine for Atherosclerosis. *Journal of the American College of Cardiology,* 64(25), 2779-2791.

Stefani, M.A., Schneider, F.L., Marrone, A.C., & Severino, A.G. (2013). Influence of the gender on cerebral vascular diameters observed during the magnetic resonance angiographic examination of willis circle. *Brazilian Archives of Biology and Technology [online],* 56(1).

Suzuki, Y., Ruiz-Ortega, M., Lorenzo, O., Ruperez, M., Esteban, V., & Egido, J. (2003). Inflammation and angiotensin II. *The International Journal of Biochemistry & Cell Biology,* 35(6), 881-900.

Tousoulis, D., Psarros, C., Demosthenous, M., Patel, R., Antoniades, C., & Stefanadis, C. (2014). Innate and Adaptive Inflammation as a Therapeutic Target in Vascular Disease. *Journal of the American College of Cardiology,* 63(23), 2491-2502.

Weintraub, H. (2008). Identifying the vulnerable patient with rupture-prone plaque. *American Journal of Cardiology,* 101(supple), 3F-10F.

Wick, G., & Grundtman, C. (eds). (2012). Inflammation and atherosclerosis. *Springer-Verlay/Wien.*

www.cdc.gov/nchs/data/nvsr/nvsr61/nvsr61_07.pdf (Last accessed November 2018)

14

THE WOUND THAT DOES NOT HEAL
Cancer

The history

Even in classical times, long before microscopes revealed what was going on, doctors knew cancer was something that invaded healthy organs. Hippocrates, the most famous ancient physician, named it after a crab with long, grasping pincers and the name has stuck. It has literally been around since dinosaurs first walked the earth because cancer-bearing dinosaur bones have been dug up. It has been found in numerous historical graves, including mummies from Egypt and Peru.

Cancer has preoccupied medical writers since they first attempted systematic analysis and some remarkably modern insights survive. The first description of breast cancer appears in an Egyptian manuscript composed over 3,000 years ago and offers the sage advice that it is a serious disease that lacks treatment. Hippocrates recognised cancer was life-threatening, and that it was caused by natural factors *not* superstitions. Galen, another ancient Greek, wrote a manuscript classifying different lumps.

Cancer has never been lost from view. The medical writers of every epoch, from classical to medieval and modern, have noted the condition and offered theories on what caused it (usually fanciful) and what might treat it (usually little). Useful insights arrived over time, albeit slowly. Gabriele Fallopius in the sixteenth century described the differences between malignant (woody, adherent to surrounding tissues) and benign (soft, mobile) masses that are observed today. He supported the consensus of ages that tumours are best left alone if possible: *quiescente cancro, medicum quiescentrum* (dormant cancer, quiescent doctor). A big step forward came when blood and lymph circulations were discovered in the early seventeenth century. This new information contradicted the prevailing view, reaching back to the humours of the classical Greeks, that cancer came from an excess of black bile. Eighteenth century French physician Jean Astruc put the bile theory to rest with finality when he compared the flavour of cooked beef with breast cancer (don't ask), and determined that cancer doesn't have bile in it.[1]

All good for a wry smile, but in many ways we are not much further ahead. We know far more than ancient physicians, and we even have treatments that work, but the incidence of death and disability is huge. Cancer kills over eight million people a year.[2] Lung cancer is the most common (also for death, as treatment often fails), followed by breast, colorectal and prostate. There are actually over a hundred cancers which can strike any organ, even the blood.

Many scientists think it used to be rare and that for the first time we are living long enough to get it. Average life expectancy in the United States was 49 years in 1900, so organs did not get old enough to malfunction.[3] Today we get elderly, so we get cancer. We are encroaching on its secrets in the laboratory, but dealing with more of

1   Faguet, G. (2015). A brief history of cancer: age old milestones underlying our current knowledge database. *International Journal of Cancer*, 136, 2022-2036.
2   Ferlay, J., Soerjomataram, I., & Dikshit, R. (2015). Cancer incidence and mortality worldwide: sources, methods and major patterns in GLOBOCAN 2012. *International Journal of Cancer*, 136, 359-386.
3   Dunne, B. (2012). Cancer. Solving an age-old problem. *Nature*, 483.

it in our lives. But there is more to it than just age — we are also doing more to bring it on ourselves.

Finding causes

Working out what causes cancer is a detective's job. You can't make people eat meat or lie in the sun to prove a point. You can watch people who do eat meat and lie in the sun but it takes decades, and you have to disentangle everything else about them. For example, the same people may smoke, drink or work in factories, so what caused the cancer, if it turns up? The difficulty is well illustrated by what the medical profession used to think of tobacco. It is now common knowledge that smoking causes lung cancer, but for many years it was far from obvious. Today, it seems quaint that a leading medical journal could say smoking only caused congestion of the pharynx,[4] or that a major study was done by sending questionnaires to English doctors who smoked in large enough numbers to make a useful study group. (And yes, it found they got cancer too). After lung cancer cases spiked upwards in the 1920s, doctors debated for 30 years whether the increase was real or due to better diagnosis; whether the excess of cases in urban areas implicated smog from factories and cars; or even whether sunshine was protective. Tobacco was on the list, but the definitive research that implicated it did not appear until 1950 in a famous *British Medical Journal* paper written by a smoker.[5] The same year the decisive numbers were published, it was still possible for a leading journal to state that for every expert who blamed tobacco another one exonerated it.[6]

---

4   Johnson, W.M. (1929). Tobacco Smoking, a Clinical Study. *J.A.M.A.*, 93, 665-67.
5   Doll, R., & Hill, A.B. (1954). The mortality of doctors in relation to their smoking habits. A preliminary report. *British Medical Journal.*, 1, 1451-1455.
6   Schrek, R., Baker, L.A., Ballard, G.P. et al. (1950). Tobacco Smoking as an Etiologic Factor in Disease. I. *Cancer. Cancer Research*, 10, 49-58.

A particular difficulty is that cancer is not a single disease but, rather, a collection of related ones with different causes and behaviours. The common theme is abnormal cell proliferation, but the science is complex and incomplete. There is a lot to be done to pin down the exact molecular mechanisms. Despite the complexity of the task, scientists known as epidemiologists, who crunch population numbers and work out which group of people died of what, have known for a long time what some of the themes are: diet, smoking and body weight. The associations are strong and widely accepted. The ones who play with molecules and work out the underlying mechanisms have been making major strides for three decades, but they still have a lot of gaps to fill. However, bear with me, and walk through the science as we currently understand it.

Role of inflammation

Cancer occurs when cells grow in abnormal ways. Instead of orderly division that maintains normal tissue, cancer cells grow rapidly and erratically. Cancer starts as a lump in the organ of origin. In time, many invade the organs next door. The last and most feared stage is *metastasis*, when tiny seeds float away in the blood to grow in distant sites such as lungs and bones.

The first insight that inflammation was involved occurred 150 years ago when Rodolf Virchow observed white blood cells in breast cancer. The most he could offer the world at that time was an intriguing clue, and for more than a century informed opinion denied there was a link. In recent decades various strands of evidence have been brought to light that converge on the same conclusion: cancer is inflammatory.

The inflammation link is so strong some authors have suggested that a tumour should be described as a wound that does not heal.[7]

---

7   Coussens, L. M., & Werb, Z. (2002). Inflammation and cancer. *Nature*, 420(6917), 860-7.

In other words, it is damaged tissue full of repair apparatus that never achieves resolution.

There are numerous heads of evidence, as per Table 1; they are of two types, which cancer authorities call *extrinsic* and *intrinsic*. Extrinsic inflammatory factors come from outside the tumour site and converge on it to turn normal tissue malignant. Intrinsic factors come from within the tissue and generate inflammation from the tissue's own genes.

Table 1

Evidence for Inflammation in Cancer

Microscopic	• **Visible inflammatory changes**
Extrinsic factors	• **Infection and foreign bodies** • **Inflammatory diseases** • **Anti-inflammatory drugs** • **Inflammatory lifestyles**
Intrinsic factors or genes	• **Tumours in inflammatory beds with no external inflammatory influences**

Microscopic

Firstly, Virchow's original observation has been greatly expanded. There are not only white blood cells in cancer but all the other paraphernalia of inflammation, such as cytokines, and processes peculiar to inflammation, such as *angiogenesis* (the process that grows new blood vessels). Blood vessels are an intriguing crossover point: new ones are a key characteristic of healing tissue but also of cancers, which need their own blood supply in order to grow.

Researchers recognise that most, if not all, cancers exist in an inflammatory microenvironment, a shell of inflammation that surrounds malignant cells and which profoundly affects their ability to survive and spread. It seems to be particularly important for metastasis, which, as above, is the term for a cancer's spread via the bloodstream to distant organs. The interaction between a tumour and its local environment is so strong that the inflammatory bed has been described as the 'other half of the tumour.'[8]

It was once assumed that cancer cells spread to distant sites because that is just what they do—a consequence of being aggressive. Researchers have now determined, by a variety of elegant experiments, that it is noncancerous inflammatory cells that cause cancerous ones to spread. Melanoma is a deadly skin cancer caused by UV light. When melanoma in a mouse is repeatedly dosed with pulses of UV, more metastases turn up at distant sites (e.g. lungs). When the primary tumours are examined microscopically, the ones with repetitive UV dosing have a marked influx of neutrophils, or white blood cells. The surfeit of neutrophils stimulates new blood vessels in which the melanoma cells float away. Armed with the findings from mice, researchers looked at melanomas in humans and found that the patients with distant spread had the highest counts of neutrophils around the primary tumour.[9]

Infections and foreign bodies

Secondly, infections can cause cancer. In 1911, Francis Peyton Rous, a junior researcher at the Rockefeller Institute in New York, published a finding about cancer that none of his colleagues believed. He withdrew fluid from a tumour in the breast of a chicken, passed it through a filter that removed cancer cells, and injected it into different chickens, where new tumours grew. In other words, he showed cancer was infectious.[10] The point was so contentious they didn't get around to giving him the

---

8   Mantovani, A., Allavena, P., Sica, A., & Balkwill, F. (2008). Cancer-related inflammation. *Nature*, 454(7203), 436-444.

9   Coffelt, S., & de Visser, K. (2014). Cancer Inflammation lights the way to metastasis. *Nature*, 507(7490), 48-49.

10 Weiss, R., & Vogt, P. (2011). 100 years of Rous sarcoma virus. *The Journal of Experimental Medicine*, 208(12), 2351-2355.

Nobel prize for it until 1966, four years before he died. We now know he was right. Cancer comes from long-term, low-grade infections that sit there like a castle under siege, not getting aggressive enough to cause illness, but not going away. The result is a slow burn which, over a long time, even decades, can turn malignant.

Viruses are particularly good at causing cancer. Rous's chicken cancer was a virus, the Rous sarcoma virus, and scientists now know of many others. These are viruses that have cottoned on to ways of disarming the immune system so they can't be cleared away, and they hang around long enough to change the environment. Cancer of the liver, for instance, is the sixth commonest cancer in the world, and the third commonest cause of cancer death. Half the cases arise from chronic infection with hepatitis B virus.[11] For a long time, number crunchers studying cancer of the cervix picked that it spread like a sexually transmitted disease and told the pathologists to go and find one. Eventually the human papilloma virus was cornered, and has been shown time and again to be responsible. In fact about fifteen per cent of all cancer comes from a long-term, viral infection of some sort.[12] And the list of blameworthy viruses continues to grow.

In the 1980s a couple of Australian researchers proposed that a bizarre corkscrew bacteria that burrows into the lining of the stomach causes ulcers and cancer.[13] They turned on its head the prevailing view that stomach ulcers and cancer were caused by spicy food and drinking too much and suggested that the relevant treatment was antibiotics, not warm milk. Doctors took some convincing, but the insight is not

11 Kim, M., Han, K., & Ahn, S. (2015). Prevention of Hepatocellular Carcinoma: Beyond Hepatitis B Vaccination. *Seminars in Oncology*, 42(2), 316-328.
12 Read, S., & Douglas, M. (2014). Virus induced inflammation and cancer development. *Cancer Letters*, 345(2), 174-181.
13 Venerito, M., Vasapolli, R., Rokkas, T., & Malfertheiner, P. (2015). Helicobacter pylori and Gastrointestinal Malignancies. *Helicobacter*, 20, 36-39.

in dispute today. Consequently, millions of antibiotic prescriptions are written every year for stomach complaints. In fact the cutting edge of research now questions whether the bacteria, called *Helicobacter pylori* for its shape, is also causing cancers of the oesophagus, pancreas, liver and colon.

It is much the same thing when foreign bodies get inside and don't move on. Bakelite was the world's first synthetic plastic (think old, black telephones) and, although it is chemically inert, if you insert a disc of it under the skin of a rat you cause cancer. Silica is a crystal in sand and rock and when industrial workers cut concrete they split off tiny floating particles of it. Millions of workers around the world inhale silica powder, which inflames the lung, a condition called silicosis. Years down the track it turns to cancer.[14] The same happens with asbestos, another natural crystal, which is sound and fire resistant and used to be popular as building insulation. The First World has stopped using it (the Third World hasn't) and is removing it from old buildings at vast expense because of the inflammatory diseases, particularly cancer, that are caused by inhaling it. Some oddball one-offs also crop up: the medical literature describes a soldier from World War II who got cancer from shrapnel fragments, and a surgical patient who got it from carrying a forgotten swab in his abdomen for three decades.[15]

Inflammatory diseases

Thirdly, some inherently inflammatory diseases give rise to malignancies as long-term complications. Inflammatory bowel disease, for instance, is a group of conditions where autoimmune factors attack the bowel and provoke inflammation. Sufferers have episodic pain

---

14   Steenland, K., & Ward, E. (2014). Silica: A lung carcinogen. *CA: A Cancer Journal for Clinicians*, 64(1), 63-69.
15   Amir, K., Malathy, K., Tashia, O., Alison, P., & Michael, L. (2014). Chronic Inflammation Predisposing to Cancer Metastasis: Lesson Learned from a Chronically Embedded Foreign Body in a Duodenal Diverticulum. *Journal of Gastrointestinal Cancer*, 45(1), 136-139.

and flare-ups for which they use powerful anti-inflammatory drugs. They may undergo surgery to remove affected pieces of bowel. In the long term, the area of bowel afflicted by years of inflammation may turn into cancer. Long-term inflammation of the prostate gland, prostatitis, increases the risk of prostate cancer. The classic yellow liver of the alcoholic, named cirrhosis, is an inflammatory state, and about eighty per cent of cirrhotic livers turn cancerous in the end. Long-term inflammatory diseases of the pancreas, gall bladder and stomach do exactly the same. It appears that the toxic products of persistent inflammation damage DNA. Damaged DNA is a mutation, and mutations are cancerous (see below).

Anti-inflammatory drugs

Fourthly, drugs that antagonise inflammation stop you getting cancer. The best known is willow bark, a medicinal substance for millennia, which Bayer AG put on the market in 1897 and called aspirin. Aspirin is a remarkable substance with multiple properties. It treats both pain and inflammation. It brings down fever. It stops blood clotting and, since the 1980s, has been prescribed worldwide to prevent heart attacks and strokes. It has also been shown multiple times to suppress the risk of cancer if taken for several years.[16] Bowel cancer is most susceptible, but aspirin also has some effect on cancers of the breast, prostate and lung. In other words, several of the biggest cancers going. Some medical experts claim that a lot of deaths could be prevented if everyone over the age of 50 and below the age of 70 took an aspirin every day. Don't rush out and buy aspirin however – it also makes your stomach bleed, and there is controversy about whether the risks are worth it. For our purposes, the point is clear: treating inflammation stops cancer.

---

16   Thorat, M., & Cuzick, J. (2013). Role of Aspirin in Cancer Prevention. *Current Oncology Reports*, 15(6), 533-540.

But aspirin is not the only option. Various drugs in the modern world block inflammation pathways and are widely prescribed for the pain of everything from sprained ankles to arthritis. Some can even be bought without a prescription. Researchers have found these drugs also suppress cancer, particularly of the bowel.

Inflammatory lifestyles

Fifthly, many different studies have proven there is a substantial link between cancer and inflammation-inducing lifestyle factors such as obesity and rubbish food.

Diet is bound up with body weight, but still exerts its own independent effects on risk. Meals high in sugar and fat induce inflammation, which is bad news for the Western world and its love of takeaways. Vegetables, fish and whole grains (not the ones turned into white flour), reduce it. No prizes for spotting which option pre-disposes you to cancer.

Roughly speaking, thirty per cent of cancers world-wide can be attributed to smoking, thirty-five per cent to diet, twenty per cent to obesity, eighteen per cent to infections and seven per cent to pollutants, including radiation.[17] These numbers are approximate, and don't add up to one hundred per cent because some cancers can't be attributed to a cause, and some people carry more than one factor (obese people smoke, for instance). There are also regional variations: in Eastern Asia and sub-Saharan Africa, where there is more of a problem with sanitation and less with obesity, twenty-five per cent of cancer deaths are infection-related. However, the main point is clear: cancer comes from things that induce inflammation.

---

17 Aggarwal, B., Krishnan, S., & Guha, S. (2012). Inflammation, lifestyle and chronic disease: the silent link. *CRC Press*.

There are some oddities. Hot spots, so to speak, of cancer in the oesophagus (the tube that conveys food to your stomach) in Iran and South America are attributed to the particularly hot beverages they like. A similar effect has been found in parts of Japan and China where people eat extremely hot rice porridge. People who live on the shore of the Caspian Sea in Iran have a cultural preference for eating their food three or four times faster than is normal elsewhere, and their staple diet is crusty bread. They too have a higher-than-average incidence of oesophageal cancer, which appears to reflect inflammation-inducing abrasion from chunks of coarse bread being wolfed down.[18] Even normal eating habits that would not upset your mother, are dangerous if your oesophagus doesn't work properly. Some people suffer a condition called achalasia, in which the muscles in the oesophagus don't relax as they should and their food gets stuck. They too get more oesophageal cancer, for the same reasons and, unfortunately, the cancer is often missed since the sensation of obstruction caused by the tumour feels just like the original condition.

These very different insights all agree with each other, and have convinced the medical world that the genesis of cancer is inflammation. The inflammatory process is intimately involved at every step from the initial tumour formation, to propagation and to the distant spread that makes the condition fatal.

Intrinsic factors or genes

Cancer is a disease of genes. Cell division and growth is controlled by genes, and cancer happens when genes get disrupted and stop working properly. The inflammatory bed, the other half of the tumour (as above), which the cancer needs to survive and spread, is not just

---

18 Wilson, G., & George, J. (2014). Physical and chemical insults induce inflammation and gastrointestinal cancers. *Cancer Letters*, 345, 190-195.

found with tumours that arise from outside inflammatory forces. It is found with almost all cancers, which means some cancers bring about their own inflammation coded by their own genes.

Genes have been recognised ever since an Austrian monk called Gregor Mendel showed that sweet pea colours could be inherited, but for a long time they were understood as abstract factors, not identifiable bits of stuff. The first suggestion they could be found somewhere – on chromosomes – came in 1914, hand in hand with a parallel insight that cancer happened when they did not work properly. A researcher called Theodor Boveri, who studied nematodes and sea urchins, suggested that genes were found on chromosomes, and cancer arose when chromosomes failed to divide normally during cell division.[19] Chromosomes, which are large enough to be seen with a light microscope, were known to be irregular in tumour tissues. We now know, thanks to Watson and Cric k, that genes are sequences of very long molecules called DNA, and a chromosome is a large rope of it. Boveri's signal achievements were showing that genes existed on chromosomes and that irregular chromosome division caused cancer.

Genes that cause cancer are called *oncogenes* and there are various ways they can get into your metabolism. Some can be inherited. We know that a tendency to some cancers, such as breast cancer, runs in families. Many of these genes have been found, and the option of getting your individual genome (all the genes that make up you) analysed to find them is not far away.

Dodgy genes can arrive with viruses. A virus can't copy its own DNA to reproduce itself, so it hijacks the reproductive machinery inside the animal it lives in, which means it sticks its genes in someone else's copier. Sometimes viral genes get left behind and become part of the host.

---

19   Seyfried, T., Flores, R., Poff, A., & D'Agostino, D. (2014). Cancer as a metabolic disease: implications for novel therapeutics. *Carcinogenesis*, 35(3), 515-527.

Oncogenes can arise when normal ones are damaged. Every time a cell divides it has to copy its genes. Sometimes the process experiences a hiccup, and produces a blip which is very different from the original. It is like multiple sequential photocopies of a picture which gets slightly fuzzier with each reproduction. These mutations, which is what they are called, can turn regular genes into dangerous ones.

Mutations can be induced by the environment. That is how tobacco smoke and radiation and many other things from sunlight to food dye turn cells malignant: they knock DNA around. Agents that do this are called *carcinogens,* and the world is full of them. One of the first to tumble to it was an English doctor called Percivall Pott, who observed in the eighteenth century that chimney sweeps got cancer of the scrotum (history does not record if he was known as Chimney Pott). He surmised that it had something to do with soot lodged in the groin, and his work led to a law that kept young men out of the profession.[20] We now know Dr Pott was right and that the culprit was sooty hydrocarbons. Around the same time another physician called John Hill made a similar observation of tobacco which, in that era, was often consumed as snuff. He warned that 'no man should venture upon snuff who is not sure he is not so far liable to a cancer; and no man can be sure of that.'[21] This warning was prescient not only with respect to cancer, but also for the role of individual susceptibility, and the uncertainty all of us carry about our own. If the warning had been heeded that long ago, the modern epidemic of lung cancer might not be upon us.

---

20 Faguet, G. (2015). A brief history of cancer: age old milestones underlying our current knowledge database. *International Journal of Cancer, 136*, 2022-2036.

21 Hill, J. (1761) *Cautions against the immoderate use of snuff and the effects it must produce when this way taken into the body.* London: R. Baldwin & J. Jackson. In: Redmond, D.E. (1970) Tobacco and cancer, the first clinical report, *New England Journal of Medicine, 252*, 21.

Many more carcinogens have been pinned down since then. Some of them are natural, like alcohol, red meat and the radiation we absorb when we go up in aeroplanes. Some of them are pollutants, such as the hydrocarbons that we inhale from things we burn. Many are synthesised, such as pesticides and dodgy chemicals that make processed food look normal. Around 100,000 new chemicals have entered the environment since the Second World War with little regulatory control, and many are suspected to be carcinogenic.[22]

Genes can be protective: Winston Churchill, famous for his daily diet of brandy and cigars, lived to be 92, yet few teetotal exercise addicts do the same. This means that some people have genes that can repair themselves when damaged, or detoxify pollutants before they cause harm, and others don't. So getting cancer when exposed to a risk like smoking is not automatic.

Obviously the question is, 'What are the bad genes actually doing?' The original view was that they disrupt the complex business of getting cells to divide in a controlled way to make a functioning organ and undoubtedly this is so. What researchers have come to appreciate in the last few years is that there is more to it. The intriguing point is that tumours always grow inside an inflammatory bed. It is this inflammatory matrix that pushes the cell towards malignancy and, once malignant, helps it spread elsewhere. It appears that a key property of oncogenes is prodding the host cell to make inflammatory proteins. Oncogenes code for cytokines, NF-кB, reactive nitrogen species and all the other familiar members of the inflammatory orchestra (see Inflammation, nuts and bolts).

The very cells turning malignant excrete chemical signals that call inflammation down around them. The tumour sits in an inflammatory

---

22 Belpomme, D., Irigaray, P., Hardell, L., Clapp, R., Montagnier, L., Epstein, S., & Sasco, A. (2007). The multitude and diversity of environmental carcinogens. *Environmental Research*, 105(3), 414-429.

bed of its own making, directed by its own oncogenes. There are multiple layers of complexity:

- inflammatory conditions damage DNA, but damaged DNA can exacerbate inflammation and keep the cycle going;

- cancer-causing viruses provoke inflammation external to the host cell by sitting there, and inflammation internal to the host cell via their own cancer-causing genes which instruct the host cell to send out inflammation-provoking proteins of its own;

- the immune system thinks a tumour, once it has appeared, is a foreign body, so further inflammation is stirred up; and

- cancer treatment, drugs and radiation may cause even more inflammation which can harm as well as help.[23]

The close relationship of inflammation with malignancy has piqued the interest of researchers. If drugs could attack the right part of the immune system would that be a cure for cancer? There are plenty of people trying to find out.

Even better, fight fire with fire. Over a hundred years ago a surgeon called William Coley noticed that patients who got severe infections in their wounds after tumours had been removed had better rates of recovery. He extracted toxins from bacteria and injected them into advanced cancers (a bit edgy, even then) and claimed to have treated them.[24] The technique never went anywhere, but he may have had a point. The immune response, tipped towards immediate attack and

---

23 *Please note* there is no suggestion that anybody with cancer should not be getting the drugs and radiation that their doctors advised for them.

24 Mantovani, A., Allavena, P., Sica, A., & Balkwill, F. (2008). Cancer-related inflammation. *Nature*, 454(7203), 436-444.

not a long-term smoulder, might help not hinder. Modern researchers are turning their minds to how elements in the vastly complex array of cells and proteins that make up the inflammatory response could be tweaked to suppress cancer rather than stimulating it. Vaccines against cancer that work by focussing an intense immune response on a specific target are well beyond the science fiction phase.[25] Some inflammatory conditions, such as psoriasis (a skin condition) do not promote cancer. That implies that psoriasis has in some way achieved a balance between good, helpful inflammation that antagonises cancer, and bad inflammation that promotes it. If the balance is possible, could human intervention replicate it elsewhere?

All interesting, but much can be done without getting sophisticated. Organisations like the World Cancer Research Fund say around forty per cent of cancers could be prevented by simple lifestyle measures like eating nutrient-dense food – fruit, vegetables and whole grains – exercising and not smoking.[26] All these measures suppress low-grade chronic inflammation. There are multiple and complex factors in play, and the science is evolving, but eating well, particularly a rich array of plant-form polyphenols, is a potent part of the equation. In the minds of some leaders of opinion, that includes concentrated foods and food extracts that maximise natural anti-inflammatory intake.

References

Aggarwal, B., Krishnan, S., & Guha, S. (2012). Inflammation, lifestyle and chronic disease: the silent link. *CRC Press*.

Amir, K., Malathy, K., Tashia, O., Alison, P., & Michael, L. (2014). Chronic Inflammation Predisposing to Cancer Metastasis: Lesson Learned from a Chronically Embedded Foreign Body in a Duodenal Diverticulum. *Journal of Gastrointestinal Cancer,* 45(1), 136-139.

Belpomme, D., Irigaray, P., Hardell, L., Clapp, R., Montagnier, L., Epstein, S., & Sasco, A. (2007). The multitude and diversity of environmental carcinogens. *Environmental Research,* 105(3), 414-429.

---

25 Dolgin, E. (2013). Cancer vaccines: Material breach. *Nature*, 504(7480), S16-S17.
26 https://www.wcrf.org/dietandcancer/recommendations-about (Last accessed November 2018).

Björn, L., Dietrich, M.B., Hubert, J. S., Holger, B., Hubert, F., & Jörg Rüdiger, S. (2001). Achalasia and Esophageal Cancer: Incidence, Prevalence, and Prognosis. *World Journal of Surgery,* 25(6), 745-749.

Bonaccio, M., Pounis, G., Cerletti, C., Donati, M., Iacoviello, L., Gaetano, G., & ,. (2017). Mediterranean diet, dietary polyphenols and low grade inflammation: results from the MOLI-SANI study. *British Journal of Clinical Pharmacology,* 83(1), 107-113.

Borrello, M., Degl'Innocenti, D., & Pierotti, M. (2008). Inflammation and cancer: The oncogene-driven connection. *Cancer Letters,* 267(2), 262-270.

Bosch, F.X., Lorincz, A., Muñoz, N., Meijer, CJLM., & Sha, K.V. (2002). The causal relation between human papillomavirus and cervical cancer. *Journal of Clinical Pathology,* 55, 244–265.

Coffelt, S., & de Visser, K. (2014). Cancer Inflammation lights the way to metastasis. *Nature,* 507(7490), 48-49.

Coussens, L. M., & Werb, Z. (2002). Inflammation and cancer. *Nature,* 420(6917), 860-7.

Cross, F., & Roberts, J. (2001). Oncogenes and cell proliferation. *Current Opinion in Genetics & Development,* 11(1), 11-12.

Deng, T., Lyon, C., Bergin, S., Caligiuri, M., & Hsueh, W. (2016). Obesity, Inflammation, and Cancer. *Annual Review of Pathology: Mechanisms of Disease,* 11, 421-449.

Doll, R. (1999). Tobacco: A Medical History. *Journal of Urban Health: Bulletin of the New York Academy of Medicine,* 76(3).

Doll, R., & Hill, A.B. (1954). The mortality of doctors in relation to their smoking habits. A preliminary report. *British Medical Journal,* 1, 1451-1455.

Doll, R., & Hill, A.B. (1950). Smoking and carcinoma of the lung. *British Medical Journal,* 2(4682), 739–748.

Dolgin, E. (2013). Cancer vaccines: Material breach. *Nature,* 504(7480), S16-S17.

Dunne, B. (2012). Cancer. Solving an age-old problem. *Nature,* 483.

Faguet, G. (2015). A brief history of cancer: age old milestones underlying our current knowledge database. *International Journal of Cancer,* 136, 2022-2036.

Ferguson, L. (2010). Chronic inflammation and mutagenesis. *Mutation Research/Fundamental and Molecular Mechanisms of Mutagenesis,* 690(1), 3-11.

Ferlay, J., Soerjomataram, I., & Dikshit, R. (2015). Cancer incidence and mortality worldwide: sources, methods and major patterns in GLOBOCAN 2012. *International Journal of Cancer,* 136, 359-386.

Katherine, E., Fortunato, C., & Dario, G. (2014). Unhealthy diets: a common soil for the association of metabolic syndrome and cancer. *Endocrine,* 46(1), 39-42.

Logan, J., & Bourassa, M. (2018). The rationale for a role for diet and nutrition in the prevention and treatment of cancer. *European Journal of Cancer Prevention,* 27(4), 406-410.

Garrett, M. (2005). Oncogenes and cell proliferation. *Current Opinion in Genetics & Development,* 15(1), 1-4.

Hajdu, S. I. (2011). A note from history: Landmarks in history of cancer, part 1. *Cancer,* 117, 1097–1102.

Hoenerhoff, M. (2015). Inflammation and cancer: Partners in crime. *The Veterinary Journal,* 206(1), 1-2.

Iyengar, N., Hudis, C., & Dannenberg, A. (2015). Obesity and Cancer: Local and Systemic Mechanisms. *Annual Review of Medicine,* 66, 297-309.

Jamrozik, E., de Klerk, N., & Musk, A. (2011). Asbestos-related disease. *Internal Medicine Journal*, 41(5).

Johnson, W.M. (1929). Tobacco Smoking, a Clinical Study. *J.A.M.A.*, 93, 665-67.

Kim, M., Han, K., & Ahn, S. (2015). Prevention of Hepatocellular Carcinoma: Beyond Hepatitis B Vaccination. *Seminars in Oncology*, 42(2), 316-328.

Macklin, M.T. (1942). Has a real increase in cancer been proved? *Annals of Internal Medicine*, 17(2), 308-324.

Mangesh, A., & Cuzick, J (2013). The role of aspirin in cancer prevention. *Current Oncology Reports*, 15, 533-540.

Mantovani, A., Allavena, P., Sica, A., & Balkwill, F. (2008). Cancer-related inflammation. *Nature*, 454(7203), 436-444.

Manuel, J. (1996). Environment, Genes and Cancer. *Environmental Health Perspectives*, 104(3), 256-258.

Nosrati, N., Bakovic, M., & Paliyath, G. (2017). Molecular Mechanisms and Pathways as Targets for Cancer Prevention and Progression with Dietary Compounds. *International Journal of Molecular Sciences*, 18(10), 2050.

Pinzani, M., Rosselli, M., & Zuckermann, M. (2011). Liver cirrhosis. *Best Practice & Research Clinical Gastroenterology*, 25(2), 281-290.

Raposo, T.P., Beirao, B.C.B., et al. (2015). Inflammation and cancer: till death tears them apart. *The Veterinary Journal*, 205, 161-174.

Read, S., & Douglas, M. (2014). Virus induced inflammation and cancer development. *Cancer Letters*, 345(2), 174-181.

Russo, G., Tedesco, I., Spagnuolo, C., & Russo, M. (2017). Antioxidant polyphenols in cancer treatment: Friend, foe or foil? *Seminars in Cancer Biology*, 46, 1-13.

Schrek, R., Baker, L.A., Ballard, G.P. et al. (1950). Tobacco Smoking as an Etiologic Factor in Disease. I. Cancer. *Cancer Research*, 10, 49-58.

Rothwell, P., Price, J., Fowkes, J., et al. (2012). Short-term effect of daily aspirin on cancer incidence, mortality, and non-vascular death: analysis of the time-course of the risks and benefits in 51 randomised controlled trials. *Lancet*, 379, 1602-1612.

Seyfried, T., Flores, R., Poff, A., & D'Agostino, D. (2014). Cancer as a metabolic disease: implications for novel therapeutics. *Carcinogenesis*, 35(3), S15-527.

Steenland, K., & Ward, E. (2014). Silica: A lung carcinogen. *CA: A Cancer Journal for Clinicians*, 64(1), 63-69.

Takeo, I. (2009). NSAIDS and colorectal cancer prevention. *Journal of Gastroenterology*, 44(19).

Taylor, B. & Waterhouse, J.A.H. (1950). Prognosis for Bronchial A. *Thorax*. 5, 257-267.

Thorat, M., & Cuzick, J. (2013). Role of Aspirin in Cancer Prevention. *Current Oncology Reports*, 15(6), 533-540.

Venerito, M., Vasapolli, R., Rokkas, T., & Malfertheiner, P. (2015). Helicobacter pylori and Gastrointestinal Malignancies. *Helicobacter*, 20, 36-39.

Weiss, R., & Vogt, P. (2011). 100 years of Rous sarcoma virus. *The Journal of Experimental Medicine*, 208(12), 2351-2355.

Weitzel, J., Blazer, K., MacDonald, D., Culver, J., & Offit, K. (2011). Genetics, genomics, and cancer risk assessment. *CA: A Cancer Journal for Clinicians*, 61(5), 327-359.

Wilson, G., & George, J. (2014). Physical and chemical insults induce inflammation and gastrointestinal cancers. *Cancer Letters*, 345, 190-195.

(2004). Letter to the Editor. *Seminars in Roentgenology*, 39(3), 341-342.

www.wcrf.org/dietandcancer/recommendations-about (Last accessed September 18).

15

KEEPING THE LIGHTS ON
Dementia and depression

The aged person who does not know her name or her children or remember anything about her life is a universal stereotype. Arguably, it is the most feared consequence of getting old. People who, in golden youth can accept dying one day, quail at the prospect of staying alive without awareness.

Dementia affects higher thinking: remembering, judging, running your life. In its mild form it means a prod to get out of bed, and someone else to cook and clean. In its severest form it means remembering nothing and nobody and every detail of living managed by others. Various conditions cause it (it is a syndrome, not a disease), and almost fifty million people suffer from it worldwide, with double that number forecast in twenty years.[1]

There is no treatment in the sense of drugs that reverse it. The literature describes sensitive ways of managing it, not drugs that cure. Numerous factors contribute, so there is unlikely to ever be a single treatment, but there is, however, a body of literature suggesting that inflammation is a significant part of the problem. The science is incomplete and controversial, but a theme is emerging. There is even a

---

[1] www.who.int/mental_health/neurology/dementia/ministerial_conference_2015_report/en/ (Last accessed November 2018)

new specialty for it called *psychoneuroimmunology* which studies how the immune system causes brain diseases.

The commonest dementia is Alzheimer's. It is named after German doctor Alois Alzheimer who studied a demented woman in the early twentieth century. With innovative stains[2] he found protein plaques and tangled nerves in her autopsied brain under the microscope; the same structures define it today. The second most common form is vascular dementia, which happens when blood stops getting through. It can happen abruptly as with a stroke, or slowly via narrowed arteries, like low power current to a light bulb.

The biggest driver is age: risk doubles every five years between sixty and eighty-five. That doesn't mean it is inevitable if one lives long enough; plenty of 100-year-old people don't have it. But the risk does go up. As we have seen (see The inflammage), a consistent feature of getting older is inflammation, and some experts see a link between the rising incidence of inflammation with age and the parallel rise of dementia. People with rheumatoid arthritis get more dementia, as do people with inflammatory conditions like obesity and diabetes. Studies that observe people over time link elevated inflammatory blood markers with dementia, particularly the vascular form, which is a neat fit with the inflammatory mechanisms that are known to silt up arteries (see Keeping the lines open). Alzheimer's patients' brains consistently show the activated microglia and cytokines of inflammation as well as plaques and nerve tangles.

There is good evidence that brain degeneration is slowed by dietary polyphenols – like those in turmeric, grapes and tea – that block inflammation and scavenge free radicals (see Nutraceuticals and where they come from). Population studies – ones that follow what

---

2   Tissues are studied under microscopes by cutting wafer-thin slices that light can penetrate. A common practice is to highlight different components by treating them with different coloured dyes called stains.

people eat for years – show polyphenol-eaters have better functioning brains after age sixty-five. The laboratory agrees: the spatial memory and object recognition of aged animals improve when fed well-known polyphenol vehicles like blueberries, green tea and açaí.

Researchers used to struggle with whether food changes anything, because of the *blood-brain barrier*. The blood-brain barrier was first spotted in 1885 by a German named Paul Ehrlich when he used a microscope to examine tissues from animals injected with a blood-borne dye. While various organs turned blue, the brain was untouched. We now know blood vessels running through the brain exert particularly tight control over the molecules they let through. For a long time researchers assumed the barrier stopped inflammation from elsewhere affecting the brain, which is a little odd as simple observations point to the reality. Illness often provokes lethargy, confusion and poor concentration – think of your last influenza – which are obviously brain responses. Body temperature goes up with illness and the thermostat for that is in the brain. Patients can lose cognition after surgery, even weeks after the event, when tissue repairing inflammation is in full swing. Obviously, inflammation gets through and, equally obviously, it is not good for clear thinking. Cytokines are very much in the frame since giving cytokines artificially induces the same changes and interrupting cytokine production prevents them. There appear to be key sites where the blood-brain barrier is leaky and cytokines can penetrate. There also seems to be a role for nerves. The vagus nerves, a pair of long nerves that run all the way down to the abdomen from the brain, can be stimulated by abdominal cytokines and carry the inflammatory message back to the control room.

In normal health, these interactions are short-lived. When the flu passes, your thinking processes recover. However, if the stimulus persists, or occurs in a brain already weakened with age, the impairment can last.

In one study of community doctor records, people who had had a significant infection in the previous five years had double the risk of developing Alzheimer's.[3] Other studies have shown older people have an increased risk if they have raised blood markers or have had a prior infection with certain viruses and bacteria.[4]

The second commonest disorder of nerve disintegration is Parkinson's disease, another condition that bears the name of a doctor. Ancient Indian and Roman authors described it (the latter termed it the 'shaking palsy') but modern interest began with an essay in 1817 by London doctor James Parkinson who described various cases including people he saw on walks around his neighbourhood. People with Parkinson's disease have a coarse tremor of their hands, a short-stepping walk and expressionless faces. We know the key is losing a neurotransmitter called dopamine in an area of the brain that regulates movement. The brains of people with Parkinson's disease have protein build-ups called Lewy bodies, as well as microglia, the hallmarks of brain inflammation. Microglia are specialised macrophages – the white cells that swallow intruders (see Inflammation, nuts and bolts) – found specifically in brain tissue. Modern research suggests the inflammation is not secondary, occurring after some other factor has caused the damage, but causative, with a caution that the picture is complicated. Some aspects are helpful: for instance, microglia stimulate dopaminergic nerve cells to sprout the multiple connections with other cells they need to function. Microglia also mop up debris that would otherwise lie around and cause harm. Unfortunately, they also release an awful lot of things you will recognise by now: reactive oxygen and nitrogen species, and cytokines. It is the familiar story.

---

3 Butchart, J.A.1.H.C. (2011). Systemic inflammation and Alzheimer's disease. *Biochemical Society Transactions*, 39(4), 898-901.
4 Schott, J. (2015). Infection, inflammation and Alzheimer's disease. *European Journal of Neurology*, 22(12), 1503-1504.

A helpful response becomes unhelpful when it outstays its welcome. But brains do not have to lose neurons to malfunction. For fifty years, doctors thought depression was a disorder of *neurotransmitters*, the chemicals that nerves use to talk to each other. When a nerve cell wants to pass a message to the nerve cell next door it squirts a spray of molecules across the gap. Some of these molecules damp down the impulse in the next cell, and some of them wake it up. In this way, impulses get suppressed or multiplied. A network of nerves firing at each other is called a brain, and a brain creates all the muscle movement, pain, emotion, personality and thinking that is you. Philosophically, the human brain could be seen as the natural world's highest achievement (but, as you use your brain to consider that, an objective opinion is difficult).

Scientists thought for a long time that depressed people feel blue because they don't have enough neurotransmitters in the feel-good parts of their brain, and antidepressant drugs were created to boost them. Prozac, probably the world's most recognised antidepressant, stops signalling molecules from being reabsorbed after they have been fired so that they linger in the gap and transmit their message for longer.

This view started with an antibiotic called iproniazid, which was developed in the 1950s to treat tuberculosis, and turned out to have the useful side effect of making people feel good. So much so, it was repurposed, to use a modern term, as an antidepressant. On limited evidence, experts decided it boosted mood by manipulating neurotransmitters like adrenaline, and the hunt for more neurotransmitting solutions was born.

In the last two decades, as evidence has mounted that inflammation is the root of many brain disorders, researchers have wondered if inflammation might be a better explanation for depression than deficient chemicals. The possibility was not outrageous, even when it was first mooted. Astute physicians have long known that depression often follows major illness, such as a heart attack or stroke. People with depression tend to have elevated inflammatory markers, and there is some evidence high inflammatory markers are a risk for suicide. Possibly it is a natural mechanism that forces us to rest up when we are sick. It is also interesting to observe that the behavioural consequences of sickness – lethargy, lack of concentration, disinterest in activity – are the same as depression. Being sick is really a minor depressive episode. There is growing evidence that inflammation drives it.

Cytokines can be administered to experimental animals to observe the effects, and to treat conditions in humans such as melanoma and hepatitis C. In both these instances, depression often follows, and resolves when the treatment ends. In one study, people with cancer of the pancreas had a significant incidence of depression some months before their cancer was discovered.[5]

Anti-inflammatory drugs like aspirin, the sort you take for a sore knee, seem to boost the effect of antidepressants in people who take them together, and a role is increasingly being recognised for anti-inflammatories in the diet. Omega-3 fatty acids, the anti-inflammatories from oily fish (see Omega-3 or not Omega-3), predispose a person to depression when deficient, and assist its treatment when given as supplements. Several ways have been suggested as to why this happens, one of which is suppressing cytokines. Several phytochemicals, particularly curcumin, have demonstrated tantalising potential in the same direction.

A question that arises is why antidepressants should work if the underlying pathology is not what everyone believed. Prozac is one of a group of antidepressants called selective serotonin reuptake inhibitors

---

5   Leonard, B., & Myint, A. (2009). The psychoneuroimmunology of depression. *Human Psychopharmacology: Clinical and Experimental, 24*(3), 165-175.

(SSRIs) which work, as above, by preventing the neurotransmitter serotonin being absorbed after it has been released. Experts are increasingly dubious about whether depression, and its cure, can be described in such a simple and tidy way.

Recent experiments have demonstrated Prozac does a few things quite independently to microglia. Specifically, it prevents calcium ions passing in – which would otherwise be the trigger for pro-inflammatory cytokines passing out – and reduces the inflammatory load generated by the microglia. Various studies have shown that treating depressed people with antidepressants suppresses the levels of key cytokines circulating in their blood.

Inflammation is likely to be at least part of the explanation for depression linked with social stress. Inflammation is higher in people caring for sick relatives, burned out in their jobs or battling at the bottom of the economic food chain. So is depression.

Inflammation is reduced with regular exercise, and regular exercise benefits people with a depressive diagnosis. Ongoing exercise, of moderate and not advanced intensity, is the most useful type for reducing both depression and blood-borne inflammation markers.

Drug developers have never found knockout drugs for dementia and depression as they are complex conditions with multiple causes. Lifestyle is no more a simple panacea than a single drug will ever be, but it is still relevant. Inflammation is a large part of the problem. Nutrient-dense plants, oily fish and the rest of the anti-inflammatory prescription, all in chapters to come, are vital tools within your hands that keep your nerve endings sparking as they should.

References

Abbott, A. (2018). Depression: the radical theory linking it to inflammation. *Nature,* 557(7707), 633-634.

Ader, R. (2000). On the development of psychoneuroimmunology. *European Journal of Pharmacology,* 405(1), 167-176.

Bahramsoltani, R., Farzaei, M., Farahani, M., & Rahimi, R. (2015). Phytochemical constituents as future antidepressants: a comprehensive review. *Reviews in the Neurosciences,* 26(6).

Brown, G., & Vilalta, A. (2015). How microglia kill neurons. *Brain Research,* 1628, 288-297.

Butchart, J.A.1.H.C. (2011). Systemic inflammation and Alzheimer's disease. *Biochemical Society Transactions,* 39(4), 898-901.

Cooney, G., Dwan, K., & Mead, G. (2014). Exercise for Depression. *J.A.M.A.,* 311(23), 2432-2433.

Dening, T., & Sandilyan, M. (2015). Dementia: definitions and types. *Nursing Standard,* 29(37), 37-42.

Desai, A. (2016). Dietary Polyphenols as Potential Remedy for Dementia. "www.ncbi.nlm.nih.gov/pubmed/27651247" *Advances in Neurobiology,* 12, 41-56. *Advances in Neurobiology,* 12, 41-56.

Felix, D., Sophie, H., Martin, K., & Ingo, B. (2013). The Blood-Brain Barrier. *Journal of Neuroimmune Pharmacology,* 8(4), 763-773.

Holmes, C. (2013). Review: Systemic inflammation and Alzheimer's disease. *Neuropathology & Applied Neurobiology,* 39(1), 51-68.

Hu, Z., Ou, Y., Duan, K., & Jiang, X. (2010). Inflammation: A bridge between postoperative cognitive dysfunction and Alzheimer's disease. *Medical Hypotheses,* 74(4), 722-724.

Janssen, D., Caniato, R., Verster, J., & Baune, B. (2010). A psychoneuroimmunological review on cytokines involved in antidepressant treatment response. *Human Psychopharmacology: Clinical and Experimental,* 25(3), 201-215.

Johnston, H. (2011). Assessing the contribution of inflammation in models of Alzheimer's disease. *Biochemical Society Transactions,* 39(4), 886-890.

Hayley, S., Audet, M., & Anisman, H. (2016). Inflammation and the microbiome: implications for depressive disorders. *Current Opinion in Pharmacology,* 29, 42-46.

Janssen, D., Caniato, R., Verster, J., & Baune, B. (2010). A psychoneuroimmunological review on cytokines involved in antidepressant treatment response. *Human Psychopharmacology: Clinical and Experimental,* 25(3), 201-215.

Keaney, J., & Campbell, M. (2015). The dynamic blood–brain barrier. *FEBS Journal,* 282(21), 4067-4079.

Kettenmann, H., Hanisch, U., Noda, M., & Verkhratsky, A. (2011). Physiology of Microglia. *Physiological Reviews,* 91(2), 461

Koyama, A., O'Brien, J., Weuve, J., Blacker, D., Metti, A., & Yaffe, K. (2012). Inflammation and Risk of Dementia: A Meta-Analysis of Observational Studies. *Alzheimer's and Dementia,* 8(4).

Leonard, B., & Myint, A. (2009). The psychoneuroimmunology of depression. *Human Psychopharmacology: Clinical and Experimental,* 24(3), 165-175.

Libro, R., Giacoppo S, et al. (2016). Natural Phytochemicals in the Treatment and Prevention of Dementia: An Overview. *Molecules,* 21(4).

McGeer, P.L., Rogers, J., & McGeer EG. (2016). Inflammation, Antiinflammatory Agents, and Alzheimer's Disease: The Last 22 Years. *Journal of Alzheimer's Disease,* 54(3), 853-857.

Mendiola-Precoma, J., Berumen, L.C., Padilla, K., & Garcia-Alcocer. G. (2016). Therapies for Prevention and Treatment of Alzheimer's Disease. *BioMed Research International,* 2016:2589276.

Miller, D., & O'Callaghan, J. (2005). Depression, cytokines, and glial function. *Metabolism,* 54(5), 33-38.

O'Donovan, A., Rush, G., Hoatam, G., Hughes, B., McCrohan, A., Kelleher, C., O'Farrelly, C., & Malone, K. (2013). Suicidal ideation is associated with elevated inflammation in patients with major depressive disorder. *Depression and Anxiety,* 30(4), 307-314.

Pathak, L., Agrawal, Y., & Dhir, A. (2013). Natural polyphenols in the management of major depression. *Expert Opinion on Investigational Drugs,* 22(7), 863-880.

Phani, S., Loike, J., & Przedborski, S. (2012). Neurodegeneration and Inflammation in Parkinson's disease. *Parkinsonism & Related Disorders,* 18, S207-S209.

Paolucci, E., Loukov, D., Bowdish, D., & Heisz, J. (2018). Exercise reduces depression and inflammation but intensity matters. *Biological Psychology,* 133, 79-84.

Schott, J. (2015). Infection, inflammation and Alzheimer's disease. *European Journal of Neurology,* 22(12), 1503-1504.

Sezgin, Z., & Dincer, Y. (2014). Alzheimer's disease and epigenetic diet. *Neurochemistry International,* 78, 105-116.

Shua-Haim, J., & Gross, J. (1996). Alzheimer's Syndrome, Not Alzheimer's Disease. *Journal of American Geriatrics Society,* 44(1).

Simone, M., & Tan, Z. (2011). The Role of Inflammation in the Pathogenesis of Delirium and Dementia in Older Adults: A Review. CNS: *Neuroscience and Therapeutics,* 17(5).

Song, C., & Wang, H. (2011). Cytokines mediated inflammation and decreased neurogenesis in animal models of depression. *Progress in Neuro-Psychopharmacology & Biological Psychiatry,* 35(3), 760-768.

Su, K. (2015). Nutrition, psychoneuroimmunology and depression: the therapeutic implications of omega-3 fatty acids in interferon-α-induced depression. *BioMedicine,* 5(4).

Wilson, C., Finch, C., & Cohen, H. (2002). Cytokines and Cognition—The Case for A Head-to-Toe Inflammatory Paradigm. *Journal of American Geriatrics Society,* 50(12).

(2014). Stimulation of Systemic Low-Grade Inflammation by Psychosocial Stress. *Psychosomatic Medicine,* 76(3), 181–189.

www.who.int/mental_health/neurology/dementia/ministerial_conference_2015_report/en/ (Last accessed November 2018)

www.pnirs.org/society/index.cfm (Last accessed November 2018)

www.parkinsons.org/parkinsons-history.html (Last accessed November 2018)

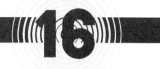

ONE RHIZOME TO RULE THEM ALL
Turmeric, queen of nutraceuticals

If a world record was calculated for the health claims made for a knobbly plant root, no serious challenger would face turmeric. Indeed, if a world record was awarded for the total cultural influence of a knobbly plant root, turmeric would mount the podium again. Millions of people have cooked, medicated themselves, and dyed their clothes with it back to eras that predate written history. Western science first noticed its biological properties in 1937, when English medical journal *The Lancet* reported that it cured inflamed gallbladders.[1] Further tentative experiments started hitting the journals in the 1970s (one study showed it was superior to steroids in arthritic rats[2]); its effects on cancer, one of its most exciting applications, turned up a few years later.[3] Since then interest has snowballed. The National Institute of Health database (PubMed), one of the world's premier repositories of health research, now lists more than 6,000 turmeric papers describing its therapeutic effects on cancer, the heart, dementia, diabetes, arthritis and the skin, to name only the most prominent.

---

1   Oppenheimer, A. (1937). Turmeric (curcumin) in biliary diseases. *Lancet*, 229, 619–621.
2   Ghatak, N., & Basu, N. (1972). Sodium curcuminate as an effective anti-inflammatory agent. *Indian Journal of Experimental Biology*, 10(3), 235-6.
3   Prasad, S., Gupta, S., Tyagi, A., & Aggarwal, B. (2014). Curcumin, a component of golden spice: From bedside to bench and back. *Biotechnology Advances*, 32(6), 1053-1064.

Turmeric grows like a flax bush. The crucial knobbly root (actually a rhizome, which propagates when divided) looks like ginger – they are cousins – and forms a yellow powder when cooked. This has yielded researchers a palette of bioactive molecules. The star turn is a polyphenol called curcumin, and two others of related shape, which are collectively known as the curcuminoids. Curcuminoids spearhead the health kick. They mop up reactive oxygen species, the drivers of oxidative stress. They have a machine gun effect on inflammatory pathways, knocking out numerous inflammatory transcription factors, enzymes and cytokines, and they are potent inhibitors of the master inflammatory regulator NF-κB.

Curcumin has demonstrated interesting effects in experiments on ageing. The best tool for studying lifespan is something that does not live very long, like a fruit fly. Various researchers have found fruit flies live significantly longer and retain markers of youth, like climbing ability, when fed curcumin. Similar results were found with roundworms, with the wrinkle that the curcumin feeders were better able to withstand heat stress and had lower levels of reactive oxygen species in their cells. When worms were bred without the genes that manage stress and lifespan, curcumin did not aid them; fruit flies with intact genes had the activity of different sets both enhanced and dampened when fed curcumin.[4] The implication is that curcumin works by manipulating the way genes are read, turning down bad ones and turning up good ones. Experiments in lower animals do not by any means translate automatically to humans, but the clues are intriguing, particularly when further evidence encompasses the big inflammatory diseases longevity is bound up with.

Heart disease, as discussed in Keeping the lines open, is caused by inflamed deposits of oxidised cholesterol in artery walls called

4 Zingg, J., & Meydani, M. (2013). Curcumin and aging. *BioFactors (Electronic)*, 39(1), 133-140.

atherosclerosis. Curcumin fed to rabbits inhibited oxidation of their cholesterol, and retarded development of the initial fatty streak, the precursor of atherosclerosis.[5] It suppressed the muscle cell and protein framework that forms around cholesterol deposits as the lesion develops. Curcumin caused atherosclerosis in mice to grow more slowly (by twenty-six per cent, compared to untreated mice on the same diet, in one study[6]); it inhibited the influx of inflammatory white cells (the ones that swallow cholesterol and store it in the wall); it inhibited disruption of artery-lining cells – disruption is the first step to cholesterol getting lodged – in arteries from pigs.[7] When coronary arteries in rats were surgically tied off to mimic a heart attack pro-inflammatory genes that would normally be active when tissue is damaged were suppressed in rats predosed with curcumin. They also suffered less damage to their heart muscle.[8] Similar observations have been made about induced strokes, which is the same event but in the brain.

A lot has been written about turmeric and cancer. Mice that are genetically programmed to get bowel cancer got less than half the expected rate on a curcumin diet,[9] and rats exposed to radiation get fewer breast cancers if they have been eating curcumin beforehand.[10] It can even help when cancer is already established: melanoma, for

5 Ramí,, & rez-Tortosa, M. (2002). Curcuma longa. *Arteriosclerosis, Thrombosis, and Vascular Biology*, 22(7), 1225-1231.
6 Coban, D., Milenkovic, D., Chanet, A., Khallou Laschet, J., Sabbe, L., Palagani, A., Vanden Berghe, W., Mazur, A., & Morand, C. (2012). Dietary curcumin inhibits atherosclerosis by affecting the expression of genes involved in leukocyte adhesion and transendothelial migration. *Molecular Nutrition & Food Research*, 56(8), 1270-1281.
7 Ramaswamy, G., Chai, H.,Yao, Q., Lin, P.H., Lumsden, A.B., Chen, C. (2004). Curcumin blocks homocysteine-induced endothelial dysfunction in porcine coronary arteries. *Journal of Vascular Surgery*, 40(6).
8 Manikandan, P., Sumitra, M., Aishwarya, S., Manohar, B., Lokanadam, B., & Puvanakrishnan, R. (2004). Curcumin modulates free radical quenching in myocardial ischaemia in rats. *The International Journal of Biochemistry & Cell Biology*, 36(10), 1967-1980.
9 Mahmoud, N.N., Carothers, A.M., Grunberger, D., Bilinski, R.T., Churchill, M.R., Martucci, C., Newmark, H.L., & Bertagnolli, M.M. (2000) Plant phenolics decrease intestinal tumors in an animal model of familial adenomatous polyposis. *Carcinogenesis*, 21(5).
10 Inano, H., Onoda, M., Inafuku, N., Kubota, M., Kamada, Y., Osawa, T., Kobayashi, H., & Wakabayashi, K. (2000). Potent preventive action of curcumin on radiation-induced initiation of mammary tumorigenesis in rats. *Carcinogenesis*, 21(10).

instance, is a nasty malignancy, which arises from the skin and which, if it spreads to other organs, is fatal. But mice with melanoma in their lungs live twice as long if they eat curcumin.[11] Prostate cancers seeded in mice had less proliferation, more cell death and fewer new blood vessels (the ones tumours make to supply themselves) after the mice ate curcumin for just six weeks.[12] In fact, there is molecular and animal evidence implying turmeric is therapeutic for cancers of the oesophagus, stomach, bowel, liver, pancreas, lung, bladder, kidney, prostate, cervix, ovary, breast, bone and blood. Quite a range. It also sensitises various cancers to conventional drugs, meaning it makes the conventional options work better.

Unfortunately, despite the promising animal data, human experiments are at an early stage. For instance, in one group of smokers with early cell abnormalities in their intestines, a high dose of curcumin for a month reduced the changes by forty per cent.[13] Other small studies in cancer patients have shown interesting effects in terms of changing key tumour molecules that imply benefit; larger studies are needed to pursue the consequences.

Another line of interest is dementia. Population research shows people in India have a four-fold reduction in the risk of getting dementia compared to the US. The reason has not been pinned down, but many researchers look approvingly towards curry. People with Alzheimer's have abnormal tangled proteins in their brain cells that slow everything down, and various lines of research show turmeric stops the tangles forming. Mice with the condition had forty per cent

11   Menon, L., Kuttan, R., & Kuttan, G. (1995). Inhibition of lung metastasis in mice induced by B16F10 melanoma cells by polyphenolic compounds. *Cancer Letters*, 95(1), 221-225.
12   Dorai, T., Cao, Y., Dorai, B., Buttyan, R., & Katz, A. (2001). Therapeutic potential of curcumin in human prostate cancer. III. Curcumin inhibits proliferation, induces apoptosis, and inhibits angiogenesis of LNCaP prostate cancer cells in vivo. *The Prostate*, 47(4), 293-303.
13   Carroll, R. E., Benya, R. V., Turgeon, D. K., Vareed, S., Neuman, M., Rodriguez, L., Kakarala, M., Carpenter, P. M., McLaren, C., Meyskens, F. L., ... Brenner, D. E. (2011). Phase IIa clinical trial of curcumin for the prevention of colorectal neoplasia. *Cancer Prevention Research (Philadelphia, Pa.)*, 4(3), 354-64.

fewer tangles when they were fed on curcumin.[14] The tangles exist in an inflammatory milieu, and turmeric stops the inflammation as well. Even people who already have dementia may benefit, although trial results are patchy. There is also molecular and animal model evidence it may also protect against Parkinson's disease and depression.

One study put curcumin head to head with a conventional anti-inflammatory drug for rheumatoid arthritis, and showed it had superior symptom relief with fewer side effects.[15] This finding is supported by various investigations which show it suppresses inflammatory biochemistry in affected joints. Other evidence shows it has promise for stabilising diabetes in animal models, and reducing diabetic complications like cataracts and kidney damage. It suppresses the low-grade inflamed state created by obesity. It alleviates diseases of inflamed skin, like eczema and psoriasis, when eaten and when used as a lotion.

There are various options for consuming it on a regular basis in order to accumulate the anti-inflammatory effect. It can be drunk as tea, boiled with rice or vegetables (which turns them golden), or eaten in curry. A key word of caution is that such methods, while not to be discouraged, are not as good as they appear because of bioavailability (see Bioavailability; getting past the border guards).

A disappointingly small fraction of curcumins get from the plate to your blood. They do not dissolve in water – which is not a good start – and they are broken down quickly once they get to the liver, so the molecules that do get through don't last. That is not to say there is no point eating it straight; the Indian octogenarians who stand out for not

---

14 Yang, F., Lim, G.P., Begum, A.N., Ubeda, O.J., Simmons, M.R., Ambegaokar, S.S., et al. (2005). Curcumin inhibits formation of amyloid beta oligomers and fibrils, binds plaques, and reduces amyloidin vivo. *Journal of Biological Chemistry*, 280, 5892–901.
15 Chandran, B., & Goel, A. (2012). A randomized, pilot study to assess the efficacy and safety of curcumin in patients with active rheumatoid arthritis. *Phytotherapy Research*, 26(11), 1719-25.

getting dementia didn't take pills, they just ate curry. And turmeric tea is a staple in Okinawa, the Japanese territory with the world's longest-lived people. It seems likely it accumulates within cells when eaten regularly, even if only tiny amounts get past the gatekeepers. There is also evidence that the crucial effect on NF-κB gene reading happens at very low blood levels, and that the molecules it is broken down into have their own anti-inflammatory effect.

However, curcumin supplements usually come with some way of upping the ante, such as hooking up curcumins with carrier molecules that sneak through the barriers. Emu oil, for instance, seems to help it along, as do emulsifiers like lecithin (the same thing that holds mayonnaise together), and even nanoparticle packaging. Another popular tactic is to combine it with black pepper since a component of pepper, called piperine, stops the liver breaking it down so fast. Piperine can increase by a factor of 20 (2000%) the amount that gets through. The technical details can be complex and don't need to be plumbed in depth; the point is that if you are persuaded to add curcuminoids to your diet for health, it is probably wise to use a commercial formula with that extra something.

References

Aggarwal, B.B., & Sung, B. (2009). Pharmacological basis for the role of curcumin in chronic diseases: an age-old spice with modern targets. *Trends in Pharmacological Sciences,* 30(2), 85-94.

Aggarwal, B., & Harikumar, K. (2009). Potential therapeutic effects of curcumin, the anti-inflammatory agent, against neurodegenerative, cardiovascular, pulmonary, metabolic, autoimmune and neoplastic diseases. *The International Journal of Biochemistry & Cell Biology,* 41(1), 40-59.

Ahmed, T., & Gilani, A. (2014). Therapeutic Potential of Turmeric in Alzheimer's Disease: Curcumin or Curcuminoids? *Phytotherapy Research,* 28(4), 517-525.

Bernard, U., & Robert, B. (2016). Is Curcumin a Chemopreventive Agent for Colorectal Cancer? *Current Colorectal Cancer Reports,* 12(1), 35-41.

Bisht, S., & Maitra, A. (2009). Systemic delivery of curcumin: 21st century solutions for an ancient conundrum. *Current Drug Discovery Technologies,* Sep;6(3):192-9

Brietzke, E., Mansur, R., Zugman, A., Carvalho, A., Macêdo, D., Cha, D., Abílio, V., & McIntyre, R. (2013). Is there a role for curcumin in the treatment of bipolar disorder? *Medical Hypotheses*, 80(5), 606-612.

Carroll, R. E., Benya, R. V., Turgeon, D. K., Vareed, S., Neuman, M., Rodriguez, L., Kakarala, M., Carpenter, P. M., McLaren, C., Meyskens, F. L., … Brenner, D. E. (2011). Phase IIa clinical trial of curcumin for the prevention of colorectal neoplasia. *Cancer Prevention Research (Philadelphia, Pa.)*, 4(3), 354-64.

Chandran, B., & Goel, A. (2012). A randomized, pilot study to assess the efficacy and safety of curcumin in patients with active rheumatoid arthritis. *Phytotherapy Research*, 26(11), 1719-25.

Chang, Y., Huang, C., Hung, C., Chen, W., & Wei, P. (2014). GRP78 mediates the therapeutic efficacy of curcumin on colon cancer. *Tumor Biology*, 36(2), 633-641.

Churches, Q., Caine, J., Cavanagh, K., Epa, V., Waddington, L., Tranberg, C., Meyer, A., Varghese, J., Streltsov, V., & Duggan, P. (2014). Naturally occurring polyphenolic inhibitors of amyloid beta aggregation. *Bioorganic & Medicinal Chemistry Letters*, 24(14), 3108-3112

Coban, D., Milenkovic, D., Chanet, A., Khallou-Laschet, J., Sabbe, L., Palagani, A., Vanden Berghe, W., Mazur, A., & Morand, C. (2012). Dietary curcumin inhibits atherosclerosis by affecting the expression of genes involved in leukocyte adhesion and transendothelial migration. *Molecular Nutrition & Food Research*, 56(8), 1270-1281.

Dorai, T., Cao, Y., Dorai, B., Buttyan, R., & Katz, A. (2001). Therapeutic potential of curcumin in human prostate cancer. III. Curcumin inhibits proliferation, induces apoptosis, and inhibits angiogenesis of LNCaP prostate cancer cells in vivo. *The Prostate*, 47(4), 293-303.

Duke, J. (2007). Turmeric, the Queen of the COX-2 inhibitors. *Alternative and Complementary Therapies*.

Esatbeyoglu, T., Huebbe, P., Ernst, I., Chin, D., Wagner, A., & Rimbach, G. (2012). Curcumin—From Molecule to Biological Function. *Angewandte Chemie International Edition*, 51(22), 5308-5332.

Gescher, A. (2013). Multitargeting by turmeric, the golden-spice: From kitchen to clinic. *Molecular Nutrition & Food Research*, 57(9), 1510-1528.

Ghatak, N., & Basu, N. (1972). Sodium curcuminate as an effective anti-inflammatory agent. *Indian Journal of Experimental Biology*, 10(3), 235-6.

Grynkiewicz, G., & Slifirski, P. (2012). Curcumin and curcuminoids in quest for medicinal status. *Acta Biochimica Polonica*.

Gupta, S.C., Patchva, S., & Aggarwal, B.B. (2103). Therapeutic Roles of Curcumin: Lessons Learned from Clinical Trials. *The AAPS Journal*, 15(1), 195-218.

Hiroshi, I. (2000). Potent preventive action of curcumin on radiation-induced initiation of mammary tumorigenesis in rats. *Carcinogenesis*, 21(10).

Howes, M., & Perry, E. (2012). The Role of Phytochemicals in the Treatment and Prevention of Dementia. *Drugs & Aging*, 28(6), 439-468.

Inano, H., Onoda, M., Inafuku, N., Kubota, M., Kamada, Y., Osawa, T., Kobayashi, H., & Wakabayashi, K. (2000). Potent preventive action of curcumin on radiation-induced initiation of mammary tumorigenesis in rats. *Carcinogenesis*, 21(10).

Jaggi, L. (2012). Turmeric, Curcumin and Our Life: A Review. Bull. Environ. *Pharmacology and Life Sciences*, 1(7), 11–17.

Jiang, H., Wang, Z., Wang, Y., Xie, K., Zhang, Q., Luan, Q., Chen, W., & Liu, D. (2013). Antidepressant-like effects of curcumin in chronic mild stress of rats: Involvement of its anti-inflammatory action. *Progress in Neuro-Psychopharmacology & Biological Psychiatry*, 47, 33-39.

Kalani, A., Kamat, P., Kalani, K., & Tyagi, N. (2015). Epigenetic impact of curcumin on stroke prevention. *Metabolic Brain Disease*, 30(2), 427-435.

Kapakos, G., Youreva, V., & Srivastava, A.K. (2012). Cardiovascular protection by curcumin: molecular aspects. *Indian Journal of Biochemistry & Biophysics*, 49(5), 306-315.

Kumar, A., Chetia, H., Sharma, S., Kabiraj, D., Talukdar, N.C., & Bora, U. (2015). Curcumin Resource Database. *Database: The Journal of Biological Databases and Curation*.

Lee, W-H., Loo, C-Y., Bebawy, M., Luk, F., Mason, R.S., & Rohanizadeh, R. (2013). Curcumin and its Derivatives: Their Application in Neuropharmacology and Neuroscience in the 21st Century. *Current Neuropharmacology*, 11(4), 338-378.

Mahmoud, N.N., Carothers, A.M., Grunberger, D., Bilinski, R.T., Churchill, M.R., Martucci, C., Newmark, H.L., & Bertagnolli, M.M. (2000) Plant phenolics decrease intestinal tumors in an animal model of familial adenomatous polyposis. *Carcinogenesis*, 21(5).

Maiti, K., Mukherjee, K., Gantait, A., Saha, B., & Mukherjee, P. (2007). Curcumin–phospholipid complex: Preparation, therapeutic evaluation and pharmacokinetic study in rats. *International Journal of Pharmaceutics*, 330(1), 155-163.

Manikandan, P., Sumitra, M., Aishwarya, S., Manohar, B., Lokanadam, B., & Puvanakrishnan, R. (2004). Curcumin modulates free radical quenching in myocardial ischaemia in rats. *The International Journal of Biochemistry & Cell Biology*, 36(10), 1967-1980. Manish, J., Shweta, S., Kala, N., Sreenivasa, S., Uday, P., M., T., V., N., & Ramakrishna, S. (2014). Improvement of Bioavailability and Anti-Inflammatory Potential of Curcumin in Combination with Emu Oil. *Inflammation*, 37(6), 2139-2155.

Mazzanti, G., & Di Giacomo, S. (2016). Curcumin and Resveratrol in the Management of Cognitive Disorders: What Is the Clinical Evidence? *Molecules*, 21(9), 1243.

Menon, L., Kuttan, R., & Kuttan, G. (1995). Inhibition of lung metastasis in mice induced by B16F10 melanoma cells by polyphenolic compounds. *Cancer Letters*, 95(1), 221-25.

Mishra, S., & Palanivelu, K. (2008). The Effect of Curcumin (turmeric) on Alzheimer's Disease: An Overview. *Annals of Indian Academy of Neurology*, 11(1) 13–19.

Oppenheimer, A. (1937). Turmeric (curcumin) in biliary diseases. *Lancet*, 229, 619–621.

Prasad, S., Gupta, S., Tyagi, A., & Aggarwal, B. (2014). Curcumin, a component of golden spice: From bedside to bench and back. *Biotechnology Advances*, 32(6), 1053-1064.

Pulido-Moran , M., Moreno-Fernandez, J., Ramirez-Tortosa, C., & Ramirez-Tortosa, M. (2016). Curcumin and Health. *Molecules*, 21(3), 264.

Queen, B.L, & Tollefsbol, T.O. (2010). Polyphenols and Aging. *Current Aging Science*, 3(1), 34-42

Ramaswamy, G., Chai, H.,Yao, Q., Lin, P.H., Lumsden, A.B., Chen, C. (2004). Curcumin blocks homocysteine-induced endothelial dysfunction in porcine coronary arteries. *Journal of Vascular Surgery*, 40(6).

Ravindran, P.N., Nirmal Babu, K, Sivaraman, K. (2007). Turmeric: The genus Curcuma. *Medicinal and Aromatic Plants - Industrial Profiles.*

Reddi, P. (2013). A Touch of Turmeric: Examining an Ayurvedic Treasure. *Advances in Anthropology,* 3, 91-95.

Shen, L., Liu, C-C., An, C-Y., Ji, H-F. (2016). How does curcumin work with poor bioavailability? Clues from experimental and theoretical studies. *Scientific Reports,* 6.

Shishodia, S., Chaturvedi, M., & Aggarwal, B. (2007). Role of Curcumin in Cancer Therapy. *Current Problems in Cancer,* 31(4), 243-305.

Sikora E, Scapagnini G, & Barbagallo M. (2010). Curcumin, inflammation, ageing and age-related diseases. *Immunity & Ageing : I & A.,* 7(1)

Srivastava, R., Dikshit, M., Srimal, R.C., & Dhawan, B.N. (1985). Anti-thrombotic effect of curcumin. *Thrombosis Research,* 40(3), 413 – 417.

Sun, A., Wang, Q., Simonyi, A., & Sun, G. (2008). Botanical Phenolics and Brain Health. *NeuroMolecular Medicine,* 10(4), 259-274.

Willcox, B.J., Willcox, D.C., & Makoto Suzuki. (2002). THE OKINAWA WAY: How the World's Longest-Lived People Achieve Everlasting Health—and How You Can Too! *Harmony.*

Willcox, D.C, Scapagninim G, & Willcox, B.J. (2014). Healthy aging diets other than the Mediterranean: A Focus on the Okinawan Diet. *Mechanisms of Ageing and Development.*

Yang, F., Lim, G.P., Begum, A.N., Ubeda, O.J., Simmons, M.R., Ambegaokar, S.S., et al. (2005). Curcumin inhibits formation of amyloid beta oligomers and fibrils, binds plaques, and reduces amyloid in vivo. *Journal of Biological Chemistry,* 280, 5892–901.

Zhang, D., Fu, M., Gao, S., & Liu, J. (2013). Curcumin and Diabetes: A Systematic Review. *Evidence-Based Complementary and Alternative Medicine.*

Zingg, J., & Meydani, M. (2013). Curcumin and aging. *BioFactors (Electronic),* 39(1), 133-140.

(2009). *Current Drug Discovery Technologies,* 6(3), 192-9.

17

OMEGA-3 OR NOT OMEGA-3, THAT IS THE QUESTION
Fish and the good oil

Of all the niches on the planet humanity has percolated into, the frozen bit at the top is the most improbable. Even if the terrain yields shelter and fire, where is the food? Vegetables don't grow there, nor do fruit or grain. A diet of whale and walrus offends everything we know about eating healthily. Indeed, it offends everything we know about eating adequately—even a hamburger has a piece of lettuce. Yet people do live in Greenland, and have done so for millennia and, once the basic tools of modern medical insight arrived there in the twentieth century and statistics were promulgated, it transpired they were doing so very successfully. When official counts were made, they found only a tiny number of the native Eskimos died of heart attacks.

In the 1970s, two Danish doctors, Hans Olaf Bang and Jørn Dyerberg, thought it was time someone from their profession went up there to find out what was going on. Fired with the spirit of original enquiry, they got themselves by dog sled to a remote spot and made the acquaintance of some cooperative Eskimos who provided blood specimens and samples of their dinner. Back in the lab, and warmed up, the doctors found that Eskimos had lower cholesterol levels than everybody else, including their compatriots living in

Denmark,[1] despite eating an awful lot of animal protein. In fact, the Eskimo blood-fat profile was markedly different in various ways.

As the researchers put it, 'Our findings might have an essential bearing on the difference in morbidity from coronary atherosclerotic disease between these populations.'[2] Their thoughtfully understated conclusion has reverberated through health-conscious circles ever since: '[The finding] is suggested... to be a special metabolic effect of the long chain polyunsaturated fatty acids from marine mammals.'[3] In other words, fish oil. They had invented the fish oil industry. Today Americans alone spend more than a billion dollars a year on pills made from bits of fish, and they have Bang and Dyerberg to thank for it. They, and the multiple other researchers who followed (there is nothing like a cool new idea for research money and thesis topics), showed that oily fish was the best thing since mother's milk for keeping your metabolism in good running order.

The magic part of fish oil is a group of fat molecules called omega-3. Omega-3 fats are the building blocks of our cell walls and our hormones, so they are important, and there are several types. Various seeds and nuts have them, but the ones from fish seem to be in a class of their own. They are the omega-3 par excellence. They have health benefits beyond the workaday business of getting cells built and hormones delivered, and a lot has been done to sort out what that might be. They drop blood pressure to a small degree, and they stop heartbeats turning erratic, a noteworthy danger in a compromised heart. They stop blood clotting (remember heart attacks are blood

---

1 Meaning the difference was environmental, not genetic
2 Bang, H. O., Dyerberg, J., & Hjøorne, N. (1976). The composition of food consumed by Greenland Eskimos. *Acta Medica Scandinavica*, 200(1–2), 69–73.
3 Bang, H. O., Dyerberg, J., & Hjøorne, N. (1976). The composition of food consumed by Greenland Eskimos. *Acta Medica Scandinavica*, 200(1–2), 69–73.
Please note that the reference to 'mammals' rather than fish invokes whales and seals but the relevant fats are the same.

clots), but probably not enough to make a difference unless you eat way too much. All good stuff, but is it enough? What omega-3 fats also do is block inflammation. Multiple studies have shown omega-3 pills soothe the joint pain of rheumatoid arthritis, or neck and back pain from spinal discs, with a greatly reduced risk profile compared to prescription pain killers. They also appear to protect against dementia. Even menstrual cramps. And acne.

Biochemists have found omega-3 fats suppress inflammatory cytokines as well as the molecules that make inflammatory white blood cells stick to the blood vessel wall. In fact, they have multiple anti-inflammatory targets in human metabolism, and new details continue to emerge. Which is all good to know if your issue is heart disease, or longevity generally, which, as we have seen, is all about inflammation.

They are also rather good for existing atherosclerotic lesions if you have any, and you do. There is less inflammatory infiltrate in the atherosclerotic lesions of people who take fish oil, and such lesions have thicker fibrous caps, which is vital as rupture of the fibrous cap is the event that causes a heart attack.

They interact with their cousins, another group of fat molecules called omega-6, which most authorities believe make inflammation worse, at least in the quantities we consume. Not everyone agrees with that, and small amounts of omega-6 are vital for some things, like cell membranes, but the suggestion is that we eat far too much. Humans evolved to eat omega-3 and 6 in equal proportions. Today we eat anything up to 20 times as much omega-6 as 3, largely because of over-processed industrial food. It seems likely our inflammatory tendencies are the worse for it. The imperative is not just to eat omega-3, but to eat less omega-6. Avoiding processed food is a good start. However, the picture is not straightforward. Initial large studies showed fish oils were beneficial; more recent ones have been disappointing. It is far from clear what the true verdict is, and various theories abound to explain the discrepancy. There are much better drugs for heart disease now than 30 years ago; maybe fish oil has been overtaken by pharmaceutical competitors. Maybe fish oil is only useful for established heart disease, not long-term lifestyle prevention. Maybe the value comes from the whole food, not a pill. For my money that one has merit. No voices dispute that fish-eaters from Reykjavik to Okinawa are better off for their habit, and repeated observations tie nutraceutical benefit in diverse forms to the complexity of whole food or its immediate derivatives. There is even a chapter in this book on it: The orchestra, not the soloist. Time will tell. The most the latest data shows is that the picture is complicated: the well-described molecular effects on inflammation and other targets are not denied; rather, the new field data is an addition to the sum of knowledge and needs to be weighed in the balance—it is not a negation of what has gone before.

Even Bang and Dyerberg have been re-evaluated. Perhaps their starting premise – that Eskimos have less heart disease – wasn't true to begin with. Perhaps Eskimo heart disease did not show up because the statistics were gathered from a scattered population who did not attend doctors when they got sick. This sort of research is like a prism: turn it this way and that and certainties blur. It is far too soon to say the whole episode has been a dead end; it is also too soon to say that marine fats are as good as we hoped.

The other snag is the quiet recognition that if fish have the good oil after all, humanity cannot avail itself of this insight because there aren't enough fish in the sea for everyone. And fish farming isn't much help, because farmed fish are fed on wild fish. Until they find salmon that eat grass, a fish farm will remain a business that turns a cheap fish into an expensive one. It would be seriously handy if fish could be left out of the equation, and minds are turning to that possibility. The fact is that fish don't make omega-3, they pinch it. Omega-3 molecules are made by algae at the bottom of the food chain. The fish eat the algae, or they eat other fish who have eaten the algae, and we eat the fish (who have eaten the fish who have eaten the algae). It all suggests someone should find a way of getting the algae to do it for us directly in a stainless steel tank so we could leave the marine environment alone. Unfortunately, it hasn't proven cost competitive, at least on a large scale, as catching fish is cheap whatever you say about the environment.

In the current state of play, one can point to major scientific authorities both for and against fish oil as a health benefit. On balance, there is no reason – excepting the environment, if that moves your health choices – not to eat seafood, particularly the oily type (sardines, mackerel, salmon), or even take omega-3 supplements, if you want to err on the side of caution, and if the arguments about the role of inflammation impress you. There is no downside: fish is not poisonous. You will be a long time catching up with the Eskimos if Bang and Dyerberg eventually prove to have been right and you had foresworn omega-3 until everybody agreed.

References

Andrew, D., Michael, B., & Terry, J. (2010). Omega-3 Fatty Acids for Cardiovascular Disease Prevention. *Current Treatment Options in Cardiovascular Medicine*, 12(4), 365-380.

Artemis, S. (2011). Evolutionary Aspects of Diet: The Omega-6/Omega-3 Ratio and the Brain. *Molecular Neurobiology*, 44(2), 203-215.

Bang, H.O., & Dyerberg, J. (1977). Lipid metabolism and ischaemic heart disease in Greenland Eskimos. *In Advances in Nutritional Research*, 3.

Bang, H.O. et al. (1977). Plasma lipid and lipoprotein pattern in Greenlandic West coast Eskimos. *The Lancet*, 297(7710), 1143 – 1146.

Bang, H.O., Dyerberg, J,. &, Hjøorne N. (1976). The composition of food consumed by Greenland Eskimos. *Acta Medica Scandinavica*, 200(1-2), 69-73.

Castrogiovanni, P., Trovato, F.M., Loreto, C., Nsir, H., Szychlinska, M.A., & Musumeci, G. (2016). Nutraceutical Supplements in the Management and Prevention of Osteoarthritis. Tegeder I, ed. *International Journal of Molecular Sciences*, 17(12), 2042.

Cole, G., Ma, Q., & Frautschy, S. (2009). Omega-3 fatty acids and dementia. *Prostaglandins, Leukotrienes and Essential Fatty Acids (PLEFA)*, 81(2), 213-221.

Deutch, B., Jørgensen, E., & Hansen, J. (2000). Menstrual discomfort in Danish women reduced by dietary supplements of omega-3 PUFA and B 12 (fish oil or seal oil capsules). *Nutrition Research*, 20(5), 621-631.

Dieter, B., & Tuttle, K. (2017). Dietary strategies for cardiovascular health. *Trends in Cardiovascular Medicine*, 27(5), 295-313.

Din, J.N., Newby, D.E., & Flapan, A.D. (2004). Omega 3 fatty acids and cardiovascular disease—fishing for a natural treatment *BMJ*, 328(7430).

Fodor, J. George et al. "Fishing" for the Origins of the "Eskimos and Heart Disease" Story: Facts or Wishful Thinking? *Canadian Journal of Cardiology*, 30(8), 864–868.

Goldberg, R. (2007). A meta-analysis of the analgesic effects of omega-3 polyunsaturated fatty acid supplementation for inflammatory joint pain. *Pain*, 129(1-2).

Grey, A., & Bolland, M. (2014). Clinical Trial Evidence and Use of Fish Oil Supplements. *JAMA Internal Medicine*, 174(3), 460-462.

Im, D. (2012). Omega-3 fatty acids in anti-inflammation (pro-resolution) and GPCRs. *Progress in Lipid Research*, 51(3), 232-237.

Khayef, G., Young, J., Burns-Whitmore, B., & Spalding, T. (2012). Effects of fish oil supplementation on inflammatory acne. *Lipids in Health and Disease*, 11, 165-165.

Leaf, A. (2008). Historical overview of n_3 fatty acids and coronary heart disease. *American Journal of Clinical Nutrition*, 87(suppl), 1978S– 80S.

Maroon, J. (2006). Fatty acids (fish oil) as an anti-inflammatory: an alternative to nonsteroidal anti-inflammatory drugs for discoid pain. *Surgical Neurology*, 65(4).

O'Keefe, J., & Harris, W. (2000). Omega-3 fatty acids: time for clinical implementation? *The American Journal of Cardiology*, 85(10), 1239-1241.

Patterson, E. (2012). Health Implications of High Dietary Omega-6 Polyunsaturated Fatty Acids. *Journal of Nutrition and Metabolism*.

Poli, A., & Visioli, F. (2015). Recent evidence on omega 6 fatty acids and cardiovascular risk. *European Journal of Lipid Science and Technology*, 117(11), 1847-1852.

Reglero, G., Frial, P., Cifuentes, A., García-Risco, M., Jaime, L., Marin, F., Palanca, V., Ruiz-Rodríguez, A., Santoyo, S., Señoráns, F., Soler-Rivas, C., Torres, C., & Ibañez, E. (2008). Meat-based functional foods for dietary equilibrium omega-6/omega-3. *Molecular Nutrition & Food Research*, 52(10), 1153-1161.

Ryckebosch, E., Bruneel, C., Muylaert, K., & Foubert, I. (2012). Microalgae as an alternative source of omega-3 long chain polyunsaturated fatty acids. *Lipid Technology*, 24(6), 128-130.

Strandvik, B. (2011). The omega-6/omega-3 ratio is of importance! *Prostaglandins, Leukotrienes and Essential Fatty Acids (PLEFA)*, 85(6), 405-406.

Thompson, A. (2013). Is the tide going out on fish oil supplements for CVD? *Prescriber*, 24(20), 48-50.

William, H. (2007). The omega-6/omega-3 ratio and cardiovascular disease risk: Uses and abuses. *Current Cardiovascular Risk Reports*, 1(1), 39-45.

Wynn, J. (2013). Taking the fish out of fish oil. *Nature Biotechnology*, 31(8), 716-717.

18

SKIN IN THE GAME (AND SEEDS)
Why the wrong bits of grapes are good for you

As far as I know, winemakers don't walk barefoot on grapes any more, even in the parts of France where making wine is a religion. The same process pertains – squashing the juice out – but imbibers no longer have to block out thoughts of ingrown nails and toe web fungus. However, the squashing bit deserves focus because it leaves behind a pile of residue, which is unfortunate. Grapes are one of the fruit world's richest sources of polyphenols, including the standout molecule resveratrol. However, up to seventy per cent of them are in the seeds, and most of the rest are in the skin and stems. Little of the goodness is squeezed out by pressing. The situation is rescued somewhat for red wine because of the trick that makes it red: juice from red grapes is clear (champagne, for instance, uses red grapes), so red wine is made by letting the juice sit with skins, stems and seeds until the colour leaches out. When colour comes out, so do the phytochemicals, many of which become the wine's character: the rough mouth-feel of red wine, for instance, is caused by polyphenol tannins. One authority has calculated that five apples, or 20 glasses of their juice, are needed to match the antioxidants in a single glass of red wine.[1]

---

1   Halpern, G. (2008). A celebration of wine: wine IS medicine. *Inflammopharmacology*, 16(5), 240-244.

Unfortunately, that does not mean a corkscrew is an aid to heart health. Possibly red wine is good for you, in small amounts, but possibly it isn't. The argument never gets settled, and factions draw up their positions around it and refuse to budge. Several decades ago it was noticed that French people live longer than their consumption of cigarettes and duck fat would justify, and many attributed the phenomenon – dubbed the French paradox – at least in part, to red wine, which the French are known to be fond of. Since then many studies have shown light drinking is healthy, and more is toxic, but there is plenty of room for argument. Studies also show a modest ongoing acquaintance with red wine reduces the risk of Alzheimer's dementia, but authorities remain cautious. Even supporters of the concept do not recommend anyone take up wine as a health food.

The obvious safe harbour is to consume grapes, not wine, but few people are organised enough to arrange a daily bunch of grapes, and even those who do will spit the pips out. There is no slow leaching of goodness from seeds and stems when grapes are eaten off the vine. What the situation calls for is some way of getting to stem and seed without a wine barrel in between, which means rescuing the discard of the vineyard press from the compost heap. Since the 1990s there has been growing commercial interest in turning wine industry waste, of which the world makes millions of tons a year, into dietary supplements. Various industrial processes boil and filter grape pressings to render polyphenol concentrates with health effects that are an exciting parallel to the better properties of wine. Such extracts are potent scavengers of free radicals; they boost the antioxidant defence system, and inhibit the enzymes that generate free radicals in the first place. They have many times the antioxidant power of vitamins C and E.

Grape extracts and grape seed powders prevent oxidative damage in laboratory animals such as rats; in one study, even rats on a high-fat diet had less oxidative stress when fed grape seeds.[2] Similar extracts modify heart disease risk in humans, even in subjects whose risk profile is skewed by obesity.

A freeze-dried grape extract applied to chondrocytes, the cells that make joint cartilage, had greater anti-inflammatory action than indomethacin, a commercial anti-inflammatory drug often prescribed for arthritis.[3]

Particular mention is due a small polyphenol called resveratrol. Starting in 1999 it was shown to extend the lifespan of yeast and flies. In mice it slows changes due to ageing by reducing inflammation, improving coordination and even fending off cataracts. Most excitingly, there is now a lot of evidence that it may delay the big-ticket items: cancer, heart disease, Alzheimer's and diabetes.

It appears resveratrol boosts sagging mitochondria, the cell furnaces that spit out free radicals and whose malfunction over time is a key connection between age and inflammation (see The inflammage). It also modifies key inflammatory bottlenecks like NF-κB. An intriguing insight is that it stimulates the same enzyme pathways as the technique of calorie restriction. Eating reduced calories while maintaining essential nutrition is a potent way of lengthening life and fending off age-related diseases. Quite how is not clear but, as always, multiple metabolic pathways contribute and resveratrol seems to feed into the same ones.

A landmark study in 1997 showed topical resveratrol prevented skin cancer,[4] and subsequent studies have extended its preventative

---

2 Choi, S-K., Zhang, X-H., & Seo, J-S. (2012). Suppression of oxidative stress by grape seed supplementation in rats. *Nutrition Research and Practice*, 6(1), 3-8.

3 Panico, A.M., Cardile, V., Avondo, S., Garufi, F., Gentile, B., Puglia, C., Bonina, F., Santagati, N.A., & Ronsisvalle, G. (2006). The in vitro effect of a lyophilized extract of wine obtained from Jacquez grapes on human chondrocytes. *Phytomedicine*, 13(7), 522-6.

4 Bhat, K. P., & Pezutto, J. M. (2002), Cancer Chemopreventive Activity of Resveratrol. *Annals of the New York Academy of Sciences*, 957: 210-229.

properties to many other malignancies. Quite a bit of evidence indicates it can slow down Alzheimer's dementia and other conditions of nerve damage like Parkinson's. It suppresses inflammation in joints wracked with arthritis.

It seems particularly effective in compromised subjects: Rhesus monkeys fed fat and sugar had less arterial inflammation when given resveratrol,[5] and resveratrol shifted the physiology of middle-aged mice on a high-calorie diet towards that of mice on a standard diet and significantly increased their survival.[6] Although evidence is mixed, it seems to reduce inflammatory markers in humans who are obese.

However, grape extracts offer many biologically active molecules, which are likely to be most effective in a team, not as individual extractions. Various studies have examined the impact of grape extracts on the inflammatory balance in humans. Results are mixed but promising, with the caveat that studies are commonly conducted for very short periods, which is unfortunate, when the postulated benefits take years to develop. For instance, one study at Queen Alexandra Hospital in Portsmouth took 32 diabetics and gave them either grape seed extract, at 600 milligrams a day, or an inactive pill.[7] The inactive pill, called a placebo, was randomly assigned without the patients or study moderators knowing who was getting what, which is a study design statisticians deem the most reliable. Everybody was

5   Mattison, J. A., Wang, M., Bernier, M., Zhang, J., Park, S. S., Maudsley, S., An, S. S., Santhanam, L., Martin, B., Faulkner, S., Morrell, C., Baur, J. A., Peshkin, L., Sosnowska, D., Csiszar, A., Herbert, R. L., Tilmont, E. M., Ungvari, Z., Pearson, K. J., Lakatta, E. G., ... de Cabo, R. (2014). Resveratrol prevents high fat/sucrose diet-induced central arterial wall inflammation and stiffening in nonhuman primates. *Cell metabolism*, 20(1), 183-90.
6   Baur, J. A., Pearson, K. J., Price, N. L., Jamieson, H. A., Lerin, C., Kalra, A., Prabhu, V. V., Allard, J. S., Lopez-Lluch, G., Lewis, K., Pistell, P. J., Poosala, S., Becker, K. G., Boss, O., Gwinn, D., Wang, M., Ramaswamy, S., Fishbein, K. W., Spencer, R. G., Lakatta, E. G., Le Couteur, D., Shaw, R. J., Navas, P., Puigserver, P., Ingram, D. K., de Cabo, R., ... Sinclair, D. A. (2006). Resveratrol improves health and survival of mice on a high-calorie diet. *Nature*, 444(7117), 337-42.
7   Kar, P., Laight, D., Rooprai, H.K., Shaw, K.M., & Cummings, M. (2009). Effects of grape seed extract in Type 2 diabetic subjects at high cardiovascular risk: a double blind randomized placebo controlled trial examining metabolic markers, vascular tone, inflammation, oxidative stress and insulin sensitivity. *Diabetic Medicine*, 26(5), 526-31.

assessed for oxidative stress, inflammatory blood markers and diabetic control. When the codes were broken, after four weeks' treatment, statistically significant improvements were found in the grape seed consumers. The results, say the authors, show grape seed extract 'may have a therapeutic role in decreasing cardiovascular risk.'

Let's drink to that.

References

Akaberi, M., & Hosseinzadeh, H. (2016). Grapes (Vitis vinifera) as a Potential Candidate for the Therapy of the Metabolic Syndrome. *Phytotherapy Research,* 30(4), 540-556.

Alarcón de la Lastra, C., & Villegas, I. (2005). Resveratrol as an anti-inflammatory and anti-aging agent: Mechanisms and clinical implications. *Molecular Nutrition & Food Research,* 49(5), 405-430.

Ali, K., Maltese, F., Choi, Y., & Verpoorte, R. (2010). Metabolic constituents of grapevine and grape-derived products. *Phytochemistry Reviews,* 9(3), 357-378.

Allard, J., Perez, E., Zou, S., & de Cabo, R. (2009). Dietary activators of Sirt1. *Molecular and Cellular Endocrinology,* 299(1), 58-63.

Anastasiadi, M., Pratsinis, H., Kletsas, D., Skaltsounis, A., & Haroutounian, S. (2012). Grape stem extracts: Polyphenolic content and assessment of their in vitro antioxidant properties. *LWT - Food Science and Technology,* 48(2), 316-322.

Baur, J. A., Pearson, K. J., Price, N. L., Jamieson, H. A., Lerin, C., Kalra, A., Prabhu, V. V., Allard, J. S., Lopez-Lluch, G., Lewis, K., Pistell, P. J., Poosala, S., Becker, K. G., Boss, O., Gwinn, D., Wang, M., Ramaswamy, S., Fishbein, K. W., Spencer, R. G., Lakatta, E. G., Le Couteur, D., Shaw, R. J., Navas, P., Puigserver, P., Ingram, D. K., de Cabo, R., ... Sinclair, D. A. (2006). Resveratrol improves health and survival of mice on a high-calorie diet. *Nature,* 444(7117), 337-42.

Bhat, K. P., & Pezutto, J. M. (2002), Cancer Chemopreventive Activity of Resveratrol. *Annals of the New York Academy of Sciences,* 957: 210-229.

Bhullar, K., & Hubbard, B. (2015). Lifespan and healthspan extension by resveratrol. *Biochimica et Biophysica Acta (BBA) - Molecular Basis of Disease,* 1852(6), 1209-1218.

Choi, S-K., Zhang, X-H., & Seo, J-S. (2012). Suppression of oxidative stress by grape seed supplementation in rats. *Nutrition Research and Practice,* 6(1), 3-8.

Dolinsky, V., & Dyck, J. (2011). Calorie restriction and resveratrol in cardiovascular health and disease. *Biochimica et Biophysica Acta (BBA) - Molecular Basis of Disease,* 1812(11), 1477-1489.

Garavaglia, J., Markoski, M.M., Oliveira, A., & Marcadenti, A. (2016). Grape Seed Oil Compounds: Biological and Chemical Actions for Health. *Nutrition and Metabolic Insights,* 9, 59-64.

Georgiev, V., Ananga, A., & Tsolova, V. (2014). Recent Advances and Uses of Grape Flavonoids as Nutraceuticals. *Nutrients,* 6(1), 391-415.

Giovinazzo, G., & Grieco, F. (2015). Functional Properties of Grape and Wine Polyphenols. *Plant Foods for Human Nutrition,* 70(4), 454-462.

Halpern, G. (2008). A celebration of wine: wine IS medicine. *Inflammopharmacology,* 16(5), 240-244.

Kar, P., Laight, D., Rooprai, H.K., Shaw, K.M., & Cummings, M. (2009). Effects of grape seed extract in Type 2 diabetic subjects at high cardiovascular risk: a double blind randomized placebo controlled trial examining metabolic markers, vascular tone, inflammation, oxidative stress and insulin sensitivity. *Diabetic Medicine,* 26(5), 526-31.

Kulkarni, S., & Cantó, C. (2015). The molecular targets of resveratrol. *Biochimica et Biophysica Acta (BBA) - Molecular Basis of Disease,* 1852(6), 1114-1123.

Leifert, W., & Abeywardena, M. (2008). Cardioprotective actions of grape polyphenols. *Nutrition Research,* 28(11), 729-737.

Marques, F., Markus, M., & Morris, B. (2009). Resveratrol: Cellular actions of a potent natural chemical that confers a diversity of health benefits. *The International Journal of Biochemistry & Cell Biology,* 41(11), 2125-2128.

Mattison, J. A., Wang, M., Bernier, M., Zhang, J., Park, S. S., Maudsley, S., An, S. S., Santhanam, L., Martin, B., Faulkner, S., Morrell, C., Baur, J. A., Peshkin, L., Sosnowska, D., Csiszar, A., Herbert, R. L., Tilmont, E. M., Ungvari, Z., Pearson, K. J., Lakatta, E. G., ... de Cabo, R. (2014). Resveratrol prevents high fat/sucrose diet-induced central arterial wall inflammation and stiffening in nonhuman primates. *Cell Metabolism,* 20(1), 183-90.

Nguyen, C., Savouret, J-F., Widerak, M., Corvol, M-T., & Rannou, F. (2017). Resveratrol, Potential Therapeutic Interest in Joint Disorders: A Critical Narrative Review. *Nutrients,* 9(1), 45.

Nowshehri, J., Bhat, Z., & Shah, M. (2015). Blessings in disguise: Bio-functional benefits of grape seed extracts. *Food Research International,* 77, 333-348.

Nunes, M., Pimentel, F., Costa, A., Alves, R., & Oliveira, M. (2016). Cardioprotective properties of grape seed proanthocyanidins: An update. *Trends in Food Science & Technology,* 57, 31-39.

O'Keefe, J.H. et al. Alcohol and Cardiovascular Health: The Dose Makes the Poison...or the Remedy, *Mayo Clinic Proceedings,* 89(3), 382-393.

Panico, A.M., Cardile, V., Avondo, S., Garufi, F., Gentile, B., Puglia, C., Bonina, F., Santagati, N.A., & Ronsisvalle, G. (2006). The in vitro effect of a lyophilized extract of wine obtained from Jacquez grapes on human chondrocytes. *Phytomedicine,* 13(7), 522-6.

Park, E., & Pezzuto, J. (2015). The pharmacology of resveratrol in animals and humans. *Biochimica et Biophysica Acta (BBA) - Molecular Basis of Disease,* 1852(6), 1071-1113.

Pasinetti, G., Wang, J., Ho, L., Zhao, W., & Dubner, L. (2015). Roles of resveratrol and other grape-derived polyphenols in Alzheimer's disease prevention and treatment. *Biochimica et Biophysica Acta (BBA) - Molecular Basis of Disease,* 1852(6), 1202-1208.

Renaud, S., &de Lorgeril, M. (1992). Wine, alcohol, platelets, and the french paradox for coronary heart disease. *Lancet,* 339, 1523-1526.

Sesso, H. (2012). Alcohol and Cardiovascular Health. *American Journal of Cardiovascular Drugs,* 1(3), 167-172.

Shrikhande, A. (2000). Wine by-products with health benefits. *Food Research International,* 33(6), 469-474.

Soleas, G., Diamandis, E., & Goldberg, D. (1997). Wine as a biological fluid: History, production, and role in disease prevention. *Journal of Clinical Laboratory Analysis,* 11(5), 287-313.

Teixeira, A., Baenas, N., Dominguez-Perles, R., et al. (2014). Natural Bioactive Compounds from Winery By-Products as Health Promoters: A Review. *International Journal of Molecular Sciences,* 15(9),15638-15678.

Tomé-Carneiro, J., & Visioli, F. (2016). Polyphenol-based nutraceuticals for the prevention and treatment of cardiovascular disease: Review of human evidence. *Phytomedicine,* 23(11), 1145-1174.

Vingtdeux, V., Dreses-Werringloer, U., Zhao, H., Davies, P., & Marambaud, P. (2008). Therapeutic potential of resveratrol in Alzheimer's disease. *BMC Neuroscience,* 9(Suppl2), S6-S6.

Yu, J., & Ahmedna, M. (2013). Functional components of grape pomace: their composition, biological properties and potential applications. *International Journal of Food Science & Technology,* 48(2), 221-237.

Yun Chau Long, T.I.B. (2014). The biochemistry and cell biology of aging: metabolic regulation through mitochondrial signaling. *AJP - Endocrinology and Metabolism,* 306(6).

19

THE GIFT OF THE MAGI
Sap of desert trees

Part of the Christmas story, and every primary school nativity play, is that three wise men visited the baby Jesus and brought, among other things, a rare gift called frankincense.[1] Frankincense, also known as olibanum, also known as boswellia,[2] is the sap of scrubby little trees from the deserts of Arabia and northeast Africa, which oozes out when the bark is slashed, and dries into beads in the sun. The harvested sap looks like yellow gravel and has been traded for millennia for its intoxicating scent – which still finds expression in perfumes and religious incense – and its potent properties as a medicine. Modern research finds much to agree with ancient wisdom. In lab rats, for instance, boswellia relieves inflammation induced by injecting chemicals and foreign bodies like cotton pellets.[3] With diseases, there is credible data that boswellia can be effective for arthritis, asthma, inflammatory bowel disease and the swelling around brain tumours, all of which, you may have spotted, arise from inflammation.

---

1 Matthew 2:11. In fact it is mentioned in various places in the Bible (Isaiah 60:6; Jeremiah 6:20; Song of Solomon 4:14), and by the historian Herodotus who lived in the fifth century BC. He recorded that the trees grew in Arabia and were guarded by winged serpents of multiple colours.
2 From *Boswellia serrata*, the botanical name of the trees it comes from.
3 Abdel-Tawab, M., Werz, O., & Schubert-Zsilavecz, M. (2011). Boswellia serrate. An overall assessment of In Vitro, preclinical, pharmacokinetic and clinical data. *Clinical Pharmacokinetics*, 50(6), 349-369.

Boswellia's anti-inflammatory properties are usually pinned on five-ringed molecules called triterpenoids, or boswellic acids, which form about thirty per cent of the air-dried resin. There are two standouts – AKBA and KBA[4] – which I mention because they get prominent treatment in the literature and in the small print on supplement bottles as the key active ingredients. It was long thought that they lead the charge against inflammation by blocking an enzyme called 5-lipoxygenase, which is not only a key mediator of inflammation, but one that becomes more active with age, particularly in the nervous system. However, more recent work shows that only tiny amounts of these substances get from the gut to the blood stream, well behind other constituents. Research shows better effects from the whole resin than the purified extracts laboratories use, which implies various elements are at work. It seems that a quite different molecule called incensole acetate, which is a major inhibitor of NF-κB, may prove to be the star after all. The point, as with all quality nutraceuticals, is to consume a preparation closely related to the natural product and its manifold ingredients to get the benefit of all of it.

Boswellia has a significant following among people with joint disease. There are many types of arthritis but inflammation, which makes joints stiff and sore, is the common factor. Osteoarthritis is wear and tear, and usually affects big weight-bearing joints like knees; rheumatoid arthritis is an autoimmune variation that inflames small joints like the fingers and deforms them over time. There are no cures, and many sufferers rely on surgical joint replacement or medications which have serious side effects such as bowel bleeds, so interest in alternatives is high. Arthritis can be induced in rats and rabbits with chemicals like formaldehyde and, when such animals are fed boswellia, it reduces the count of white

4   Acetyl-11-keto-β-boswellic acid and 11-keto-β-boswellic acid.

blood cells inside their joints and resolves lameness. When arthritic rat joints are sliced and examined under a microscope, those treated with boswellia show less bone death and joint erosion.[5] Results from trials with people are mixed but, taken overall, they point towards efficacy with far less toxicity than mainstream medicines, particularly for osteoarthritis. In trials that compare boswellia with a placebo, people with osteoarthritis have statistically significant improvements in joint function and reduction in pain.[6]

The gut is another seat of chronic inflammation for some unlucky people. Conditions like Crohn's disease inflict years of pain and bleeding and render patients dependent on powerful drugs, like steroids, for relief. Experiments that induce artificial inflammation in rat guts show boswellia stops white blood cells sticking to blood vessel walls, an essential step in inflammation, with an efficacy comparable to conventional medication.[7]

It also seems to help the gut lining hold together in the face of inflammatory onslaught. The lining of the gut is a single layer of tightly bound cells which keeps out toxins and bacteria and regulates what gets absorbed. It breaks down when inflamed. After their guts were inflamed with noxious chemicals, mice maintained their gut linings in watertight condition when dosed with boswellia.[8]

The leading study of actual Crohn's patients, as opposed to poisoned mice, showed no difference between patients treated with boswellia, and ones treated with a conventional drug called mesalazine. In other

5 Umar, S., Umar, K., Sarwar, A., Khan, A., Ahmad, N., Ahmad, S., Katiyar, C., Husain, S., & Khan, H. (2014). Boswellia serrata extract attenuates inflammatory mediators and oxidative stress in collagen induced arthritis. *Phytomedicine*, 21(6), 847-856.
6 Grover, A.K., & Samson, S.E. (2015). Benefits of antioxidant supplements for knee osteoarthritis: rationale and reality. *Nutrition Journal*. 15(1).
7 Abdel-Tawab, M., Werz, O., & Schubert-Zsilavecz, M. (2011). Boswellia serrate. An overall assessment of In Vitro, preclinical, pharmacokinetic and clinical data. *Clinical Pharmacokinetics*, 50(6), 349-369.
8 Catanzaro, D., Rancan, S., Orso, G., et al. (2015). Boswellia serrata: Preserves Intestinal Epithelial Barrier from Oxidative and Inflammatory Damage. Deli MA, ed. *PLoS ONE*. 10(5).

words, boswellia performed as well as mesalazine did.[9] Data on boswellia in asthma (airway inflammation) is limited, but one study that compared boswellia with placebo produced statistically significant improvements in lung function in asthma sufferers.[10] There is indirect evidence it stabilises mast cells, specialised inflammatory cells that produce histamine, which is a potent mediator of the allergies and airway constriction that characterises asthma.

And finally, brain tumours. Inflammation around cancer causes swelling. When cancer lodges in the brain the swelling is a distinct problem, because the brain lives inside a rigid box and is particularly sensitive to being squashed. Unfortunately, radiotherapy, one of the major brain tumour treatments, makes the swelling worse. Swelling aggravates brain tumour symptoms like loss of function and patients often need steroids to stay on top of it. One study randomly split forty-four brain tumour patients between boswellia and placebo treatments as they underwent radiotherapy; sixty per cent of the boswellia patients reduced their swelling by over three quarters, and only twenty-six per cent of the others did.[11] Other studies, albeit with small numbers of people, have had similar results. Even more exciting is the observation that boswellia kills cancer cells grown in test media and leaves normal cells alone. Cancers of the breast and pancreas, among others, have been seen to succumb to boswellia treatment in the laboratory. As is so often the case with promising nutraceuticals, trials in humans have yet to be done, but indications are that boswellia could be a major agent for multiple different malignancies.

9   Gerhardt, H., Seifert, F., Buvari, P., Vogelsang, H., & Repges, R. (2001). Therapy of active Crohn disease with Boswellia serrata extract H 15. Z Gastroenterology. 39(1), 11-7 [Article in German].

10 Gupta, I., Gupta, V., Parihar, A., Gupta, S., Lüdtke, R., Safayhi, H., & Ammon, H.P. (1998). Effects of Boswellia serrata gum resin in patients with bronchial asthma: results of a double-blind, placebo-controlled, 6-week clinical study. European Journal of Medical Research, 3(11), 511-4.

11 Kirste, S., Treier, M., Wehrle, S.J., Becker, G., Abdel-Tawab, M., Gerbeth, K., Hug, M.J., Lubrich, B., Grosu, A.L., & Momm, F.(2011). Boswellia serrata acts on cerebral edema in patients irradiated for brain tumors: a prospective, randomized, placebo-controlled, double-blind pilot trial. Cancer. 117(16), 3788-95.

To complete the picture, boswellia appears to cause few side effects, even at high doses. Occasional minor gastrointestinal upset seems to be the only issue, which is remarkable compared to the substantial and lethal side effects mainstream anti-inflammatories are capable of.

References

Abdel-Tawab, M., Werz, O., & Schubert-Zsilavecz, M. (2011). Boswellia serrate. An overall assessment of In Vitro, preclinical, pharmacokinetic and clinical data. *Clinical Pharmacokinetics,* 50(6), 349-369.

Ahmed, H.H., Abd-Rabou, A.A., & Hassan, A.Z. (2015). Phytochemical Analysis and Anti-cancer Investigation of Boswellia serrata Bioactive Constituents In Vitro. *Asian Pacific Journal of Cancer Prevention,* 16(16), 7179-88.

Ammon, H.P.T., Safayhi, H, Mack, T. & Sabieraj, J. (1993). Mechanism of antiinflammatory actions of curcumine and boswellic acids. *Journal of Ethnopharmacology,* 38.

Catanzaro, D., Rancan, S., Orso, G., et al. (2015). Boswellia serrata: Preserves Intestinal Epithelial Barrier from Oxidative and Inflammatory Damage. Deli MA, ed. *PLoS ONE,* 10(5).

Cerutti-Delasalle, C., Mehiri, M., Cagliero, C., Rubiolo, P., Bicchi, C., Meierhenrich, U., & Baldovini, N. (2017). The (+)-cis- and (+)-trans-Olibanic Acids: Key Odorants of Frankincense. *Angewandte Chemie,* 128(44), 13923-13927.

Gerhardt, H., Seifert, F., Buvari, P., Vogelsang, H., & Repges, R. (2001). Therapy of active Crohn disease with Boswellia serrata extract H 15. *Z Gastroenterology,* 39(1), 11-7 [Article in German].

Grover, A.K., & Samson, S.E. (2015). Benefits of antioxidant supplements for knee osteoarthritis: rationale and reality. *Nutrition Journal,* 15(1).

Gupta, I., Gupta, V., Parihar, A., Gupta, S., Lüdtke, R., Safayhi, H., & Ammon, H.P. (1998). Effects of Boswellia serrata gum resin in patients with bronchial asthma: results of a double-blind, placebo-controlled, 6-week clinical study. *European Journal of Medical Research,* 3(11), 511-4.

Kirste, S., Treier, M., Wehrle, S.J., Becker, G., Abdel-Tawab, M., Gerbeth, K., Hug, M.J., Lubrich, B., Grosu, A.L., & Momm, F.(2011). Boswellia serrata acts on cerebral edema in patients irradiated for brain tumors: a prospective, randomized, placebo-controlled, double-blind pilot trial. *Cancer,* 117(16), 3788-95.

Moussaieff, A., & Mechoulam, R. (2009). Boswellia resin: from religious ceremonies to medical uses; a review of in-vitro, in-vivo and clinical trials. *Journal of Pharmacy and Pharmacology: An International Journal of Pharmaceutical Science,* 61(10).

Ni, X., Suhail, M., Yang, Q., et al. (2012). Frankincense essential oil prepared from hydrodistillation of Boswellia Sacra gum resins induces human pancreatic cell death in cultures and in a xenograft murine model. *BMC Complementary and Alternative Medicine,* 12,253.

Suhail, M., Weijuan, W., Cao, A., et al. (2011). Boswellia sacra essential oil induces tumor cell specific apoptosis and suppresses tumour aggressiveness in cultured human breast cancer cells. *BMC Complementary and Alternative Medicine,* 11(129).

Umar, S., Umar, K., Sarwar, A., Khan, A., Ahmad, N., Ahmad, S., Katiyar, C., Husain, S., & Khan, H. (2014). Boswellia serrata extract attenuates inflammatory mediators and oxidative stress in collagen induced arthritis. *Phytomedicine*, 21(6), 847-856.

Zhang, Y., Ning, Z., Lu, C., Zhao, S., Wang, J., Liu, B., Xu, X., & Liu, Y. (2013). Triterpenoid resinous metabolites from the genus Boswellia: pharmacological activities and potential species-identifying properties. *Chemistry Central Journal*, 7(1), 1-16.

(2008) Chemical & Engineering News, 86(51)

20

THE FIRE IN THE FAT
The good and bad bits of body bulges

If you look at fat cells down a microscope, you see a thin-walled lattice like chicken wire with white blobs inside. The white blobs are fat, which stores energy. Fat stores were vital when humans lived by the seasons for food, but today we eat more energy than we need, and the storage arrangements are problematic. Doctors have known for a long time that too much fat in your make-up goes with heart disease, diabetes and cancer, particularly breast and bowel – even dementia – although at first glance it is not obvious why.

The associations were thrown up by population studies, but a cause-and-effect mechanism was never obvious because everyone thought fat cells (called adipocytes) were passive deposits, like a fuel depot. Turns out, they aren't. In 1994, researchers for the first time isolated an immune-modulating cytokine (see <u>Inflammation, nuts and bolts</u>) made by fat tissue. Called leptin, it regulates body weight, among many other things, and the receptors it acts on appear in diverse tissues including the white blood cells of the immune system. Since then it has been shown that fat tissue makes more than six hundred other metabolically active molecules which float away and manipulate your physiology at distant sites. Key among these are inflammatory cytokines, which have even been given their own word—*adipokines*.

The bridge between fat and disease is largely inflammation. Fat is not a depot, it is a signalling station. There is even a new academic field for it—*immunometabolism*.

Obese people have elevated inflammatory proteins in their blood, and fat tissue is routinely infiltrated by inflammatory white blood cells. So much so that researchers – exasperated with poor results from traditional diet advice – now wonder if the key treatment for obesity is not better weight loss drugs, but ones that block adipokines. In other words, the fat would be manageable if the messages it sends could be stopped. The concept is interesting, but well short of commercial release, so do not anticipate discarding the conventional approach any time soon.

Everybody has adipocytes, but in overweight people they are stretched, like bulging suitcases, and it is these that are inflammatory. Fat cells can vary in size by a factor of 10, depending on how much is squashed into them, and bulging cells function poorly. Their DNA turns hypermethylated (see Epigenetics, and food as information) which skews it towards inflammatory functions. They die and release debris and white blood cells move in to clear the site. In obesity anything up to half of the cells in fat tissue are the blood-derived cells of inflammation. It is these foot soldiers, recruited to keep order, whose cytokines flood the body.

Obesity is commonly calculated via the Body Mass Index (BMI), which is a universally recognised formula that compares height to weight. It is simple and effective, but it can be misleading. Muscular athletes can come out as obese, for instance. BMI only approximates crudely to your fat content. Not only that, BMI does not tell you what sort of fat you have.

That matters because not all fat is created equal. Fat under your skin – by far the most abundant type – is fairly benign, particularly on the lower body. Big thighs are not a worry (which, incidentally, means, liposuction doesn't make you healthier even if it makes you less fat).

Fat around the organs in your abdomen, so called visceral fat, is dangerous; it is a reason doctors emphasise girth size, particularly for men. A degree of abdominal packing fat is normal, but the risk goes up sharply when normal levels are exceeded.

The most ominous deposits are 'ectopic' ones, which is fat where it is not meant to be, like inside the liver and around the heart. A fatty liver, for instance, is a bigger risk for heart disease than smoking, high blood pressure or diabetes.[1]

Some experts suggest that BMI is less useful than ratios of waist-to-hip or waist-to-height, which better capture fat distribution. Lean people with pot bellies (the metabolically obese) share the inflammatory risks of the overweight. Likewise, some obese people can be metabolically healthy if their fat is in the right place.

Generally excess energy prefers your skin sites, and only spills into the abdomen when they are saturated. Quite possibly that is part of why abdominal fat is dangerous; it signals you are eating more than your body is designed to hold, like water over the top of a dam. And too much food means too many reactive oxygen species when you burn it, as per The inflammage. It also appears that unremitting food deliveries gum up the ebb and flow of energy that mitochondria were designed for and exhausts them. Worn out mitochondria are another potent force in tissue ageing.

So total fat is not so much the health issue as where, and the difference appears to come down to inflammatory behaviour. Abdominal and ectopic fat, for whatever reason, engage the inflammatory mechanisms more aggressively than skin deposits. It is also plausible that adipokines

---

1   DiNicolantonio, J., Lucan, S., & O'Keefe, J. (2016). The Evidence for Saturated Fat and for Sugar Related to Coronary Heart Disease. *Progress in Cardiovascular Diseases*, 58(5), 464-472.

made by fat next door to vital organs attack them with more vigour than ones that float in from distant sites.

Food with added sugar appears to aggravate visceral fat, as does processed food generally, along with personal stress and alcohol. Fibre in vegetables, particularly beans, improves it. Well-known systems of healthy eating like the Mediterranean diet also improve it. And possibly there is more to it than energy: tentative evidence suggests the antioxidant phytochemicals in healthy diets play a part.[2]

Unfortunately, time drives it too. As decades pass your metabolism changes, and more and more fat slips into your abdomen. Many readers of this book will nod in quiet recognition.

The good news is that dangerous fat is first to leave when asked. Healthy eating and exercise have the greatest effect on the worst deposits. Crucially, this means that body weight, although important, is not a reliable guide to how much good the right lifestyle choices are doing. Many of the health-conscious middle-aged despair when the morning scales do not recognise their efforts, but weight is not the only weighty consideration. The point is where, not just how much, and the scales do not tell you.

In one major recent study in Israel, participants adopted the Mediterranean diet, and were monitored with body scans.[3] The ectopic deposits melted away. The Mediterranean diet is not short on fat – certain fish like sardines are fatty, as is olive oil – but the diet removed ectopics better than a low-fat alternative did. The major conclusion of the study designers, to the delight of frustrated dieters

---

2 Mechanick, J., Zhao, S., & Garvey, W. (2016). The Adipokine-Cardiovascular-Lifestyle Network. *Journal of the American College of Cardiology*, 68(16), A1-A38.

3 Gepner, Y., Shelef, I., Schwarzfuchs, D., Zelicha, H., Tene, L., Yaskolka Meir, A., Tsaban, G., Cohen, N., Bril, N., Rein, M., Serfaty, D., Kenigsbuch, S., Komy, O., Wolak, A., Chassidim, Y., Golan, R., Avni-Hassid, H., Bilitzky, A., Sarusi, B., Goshen, E., Shemesh, E., Henkin, Y., Stumvoll, M., Blüher, M., Thiery, J., Ceglarek, U., Rudich, A., Stampfer, M., & Shai, I. (2018). Effect of Distinct Lifestyle Interventions on Mobilization of Fat Storage Pools. *Circulation*, 137(11), 1143-1157.

worldwide, is that modest weight loss from eating well underestimates the significant benefits on fat distribution. Other research has found the same.

Likewise, modest exercise mobilises visceral fat first. Modest exercise is often advocated as a life-extending, inflammation-damping lifestyle tool (see Run for your life), and its precision attack on your most dangerous fat is part of the reason.

So keep walking and eating well, and add healthy fat allocation to the list of the anti-inflammatory payoffs.

References

Boutens, L., & Stienstra, R. (2016). Adipose tissue macrophages: going off track during obesity. *Diabetologia*, 59, 879-894.

Cao, Q., Yu, S., Xiong, W., et al. (2018). Waist-hip ratio as a predictor of myocardial infarction risk: A systematic review and meta-analysis. Chattipakorn, N., ed. *Medicine*, 97(30).

Cleal, L., Aldea, T., & Chau, Y-Y. (2017). Fifty shades of white: Understanding heterogeneity in white adipose stem cells. *Adipocyte*, 6(3), 205-216.

Deng, T., Lyon, C., Bergin, S., Caligiuri, M., & Hsueh, W. (2016). Obesity, Inflammation, and Cancer. *Annual Review of Pathology: Mechanisms of Disease*, 11, 421-449.

Eheim, A., Medrikova, D., & Herzig, S. (2013). Immune cells and metabolic dysfunction. *Seminars in Immunopathology*, 36(1), 13-25.

Finelli, C., Sommella, L., Gioia, S., La Sala, N., & Tarantino, G. (2013). Should visceral fat be reduced to increase longevity? *Ageing Research Reviews*, 12(4), 996-1004.

Farb, M.G., & Gokce, N. (2015). Visceral adiposopathy: a vascular perspective. *Hormone Molecular Biology and Clinical Investigation*, 21(2), 125-136.

Finelli, C., Sommella, L., Gioia, S., La Sala, N., & Tarantino, G. (2013). Should visceral fat be reduced to increase longevity? *Ageing Research Reviews*, 12(4), 996-1004.

Francisco, V., Pino, J., Gonzalez-Gay, M., Mera, A., Lago, F., Gómez, R., Mobasheri, A., & Gualillo, O. (2018). Adipokines and inflammation: is it a question of weight? *British Journal of Pharmacology*, 175(10), 1569-1579.

Gepner, Y., Shelef, I., Schwarzfuchs, D., Zelicha, H., Tene, L., Yaskolka Meir, A., Tsaban, G., Cohen, N., Bril, N., Rein, M., Serfaty, D., Kenigsbuch, S., Komy, O., Wolak, A., Chassidim, Y., Golan, R., Avni-Hassid, H., Bilitzky, A., Sarusi, B., Goshen, E., Shemesh, E., Henkin, Y., Stumvoll, M., Blüher, M., Thiery, J., Ceglarek, U., Rudich, A., Stampfer, M., & Shai, I. (2018). Effect of Distinct Lifestyle Interventions on Mobilization of Fat Storage Pools. *Circulation*, 137(11), 1143-1157.

Gilbert, C., & Slingerland, J. (2013). Cytokines, Obesity, and Cancer: New Insights on Mechanisms Linking Obesity to Cancer Risk and Progression. *Annual Review of Medicine*, 64, 45-57.

Goss, A., Goree, L., Ellis, A., Chandler-Laney, P., Casazza, K., Lockhart, M., & Gower, B. (2013). Effects of diet macronutrient composition on body composition and fat distribution during weight maintenance and weight loss. *Obesity*, 21(6), 1139-1142.

Hill, J., Solt, C., & Foster, M. (2018). Obesity associated disease risk: the role of inherent differences and location of adipose depots. *Hormone Molecular Biology and Clinical Investigation*, 33(2).

Hughes-Austin, J., Larsen, B., & Allison, M. (2013). Visceral Adipose Tissue and Cardiovascular Disease Risk. *Current Cardiovascular Risk Reports*, 7(2), 95-101.

Iacobellis, G., & Barbaro, G. (2018). Targeting the organ-specific adiposity. Eating and Weight Disorders - Studies on Anorexia, Bulimia and Obesity, *OnlineFirst*.

Iyengar, N., Hudis, C., & Dannenberg, A. (2015). Obesity and Cancer: Local and Systemic Mechanisms. *Annual Review of Medicine*, 66, 297-309.

Jemtel, T., Samson, R., Milligan, G., Jaiswal, A., & Oparil, S. (2018). Visceral Adipose Tissue Accumulation and Residual Cardiovascular Risk. *Current Hypertension Reports*, 20(9), 1-14.

Kelli, H., Corrigan, F., Heinl, R., Dhindsa, D., Hammadah, M., Samman-Tahhan, A., Sandesara, P., O'Neal, W., Al Mheid, I., Ko, Y., Vaccarino, V., Ziegler, T., Sperling, L., Brigham, K., Jones, D., Martin, G., & Quyyumi, A. (2017). Relation of Changes in Body Fat Distribution to Oxidative Stress. *The American Journal of Cardiology*, 120(12), 2289-2293.

Kim, M., Tanaka, K., Kim, M., Matuso, T., Endo, T., Tomita, T., Maeda, S., & Ajisaka, R. (2009). Comparison of epicardial, abdominal and regional fat compartments in response to weight loss. *Nutrition, Metabolism and Cardiovascular Diseases*, 19(11), 760-766.

Klein, M., & Varga, I. (2018). Microenvironment of Immune Cells Within the Visceral Adipose Tissue Sensu Lato vs. Epicardial Adipose Tissue: What Do We Know? *Inflammation*, 41(4), 1142-1156.

Klöting, N., & Blüher, M. (2014). Adipocyte dysfunction, inflammation and metabolic syndrome. *Reviews in Endocrine and Metabolic Disorders*, 15(4), 277-287.

Lettieri Barbato, D., & Aquilano, K. (2016). Feast and famine: Adipose tissue adaptations for healthy aging. *Ageing Research Reviews*, 28, 85-93.

Ma, J., Karlsen, M.C., Chung, M., et al. (2016). Potential link between excess added sugar intake and ectopic fat: a systematic review of randomized controlled trials. *Nutrition Reviews*, 74(1), 18-32.

Manno, C., Campobasso, N., Nardecchia, A., Triggiani, V., Zupo, R., Gesualdo, L., Silvestris, F., & Pergola, G. (2018). Relationship of para- and perirenal fat and epicardial fat with metabolic parameters in overweight and obese subjects. Eating and Weight Disorders - Studies on Anorexia, Bulimia and Obesity, *OnlineFirst*, 1-6.

Mau, T., & Yung, R. (2018). Adipose tissue inflammation in aging. *Experimental Gerontology*, 105, 27-31.

Mechanick, J., Zhao, S., & Garvey, W. (2016). The Adipokine-Cardiovascular-Lifestyle Network. *Journal of the American College of Cardiology*, 68(16), A1-A38.

Mercer, J., Hoggard, N., & Morgan, P. (2012). Leptin and Obesity. *CNS Drugs*, 14(6), 413-424.

Motamed, N., Perumal, D., Zamani, F., Ashrafi, H., Haghjoo, M., Saeedian, F., Maadi, M., Akhavan-Niaki,

H., Rabiee, B., & Asouri, M. (2015). Conicity Index and Waist-to-Hip Ratio Are Superior Obesity Indices in Predicting 10-Year Cardiovascular Risk Among Men and Women. *Clinical Cardiology,* 38(9), 527-534.

O'Rourke, R. (2009). Inflammation in obesity-related diseases. *Surgery,* 145(3), 255-259.

Palmer, A., & Kirkland, J. (2016). Aging and adipose tissue: potential interventions for diabetes and regenerative medicine. *Experimental Gerontology,* 86, 97-105.

Pararasa, C., Bailey, C., & Griffiths, H. (2014). Ageing, adipose tissue, fatty acids and inflammation. *Biogerontology,* 16(2), 235-248

Park, Y.J., Park, J., Huh, J.Y., Hwang, I., Choe, S.S., & Kim, J.B. (2018). Regulatory Roles of Invariant Natural Killer T Cells in Adipose Tissue Inflammation: Defenders Against Obesity-Induced Metabolic Complications. *Frontiers in Immunology,* 9 :10.3389/fimmu.2018.01311.

Pilolla, K. (2018). Targeting abdominal obesity through the diet. *ACSM's Health & Fitness Journal,* 22(5), 21-28.

Sam, S. (2018). Differential effect of subcutaneous abdominal and visceral adipose tissue on cardiometabolic risk. *Hormone Molecular Biology and Clinical Investigation,* 33(1).

Smith, U., & Hammarstedt, A. (2010). Antagonistic effects of thiazolidinediones and cytokines in lipotoxicity. Biochimica et Biophysica Acta (BBA), *Molecular and Cell Biology of Lipids,* 1801(3), 377-380.

Walker, G., Marzullo, P., Ricotti, R., Bona, G., & Prodam, F. (2014). The pathophysiology of abdominal adipose tissue depots in health and disease. *Hormone Molecular Biology and Clinical Investigation,* 19(1).

21

AN OLIVE BRANCH
How the wrong bits of olive trees are good for you

Put extra virgin olive oil in a glass and throw it back like a shot of Scotch and it will burn your throat. Scientists used to be puzzled by that. Olive oil is rich and unctuous, so where does the spicy backbone come from? Nobody knew until 2003, when food scientists found oleocanthal (*oleo* = olive and *canth* = sting). It proved to be a significant discovery, because oleocanthal does not just transmit flavour, it also turns out to be a potent anti-inflammatory. In fact, it is so powerful it blocks inflammatory enzymes as well as a commercial drug called ibuprofen, which doctors prescribe for inflammatory conditions like arthritis.[1]

Until recently, scientists thought they knew where they were with olive oil: it lubricates all the cuisines around the Mediterranean Sea, and the Mediterranean diet – a classic package of vegetables, fish and occasional wine – is well known to deliver health and long life. Olive oil is widely accepted as a large part of the benefit, but experts have recently had to rethink how it works.

1 Beauchamp, G.K., Russell, N., Keast, S.J., Morel, D., Lin, J., Pika, J., Han, Q., Lee, C-H., Smith, A.B., & Paul, A.S. (2005). Breslin Ibuprofen-like activity in extra-virgin olive oil. *Nature*, 437, 45–46.

For some time, dietary advice drew a sharp distinction between saturated fat,[2] most of which (like milk and meat) is sourced from animals, and the unsaturated alternative from plants like nuts and seeds. Unsaturated was healthier. Olive oil is mainly an unsaturated fat called oleic acid, so the long-life payoff was easy to explain. However, the saturated and unsaturated distinction is starting to look dubious. Modern studies show it is no longer possible to confidently state one is superior,[3] which implies olive oil must be helpful on some other front. As a whole food, olive oil contains numerous micronutrients, particularly polyphenols, which are increasingly drawing attention as the real source of the health kick. It illustrates a problem that permeates fat advice generally: definitions based on broad classes of fat forget that whole food is made of multiple ingredients, each with health benefits of their own. There is more to healthy eating than counting macronutrients.

A major Spanish study of more than 7,000 people at high risk of heart disease showed that the Mediterranean diet, supplemented with extra olive oil or nuts, significantly reduced heart disease,[4] and was more effective than an alternative diet that emphasised reduced fat. Subsequent work showed that the benefit was correlated with total polyphenols, particularly lignans, which are potent antioxidants.

---

2 Fats are chains of carbon atoms. Saturated ones have single bonds between their atoms and therefore have less ability to form reactions with other molecules. Unsaturated fats have one or more double bonds, which can be broken and reformed with other molecules without disrupting the chain (monounsaturated have one double bond, polyunsaturated have more). A useful rule of thumb is that saturated fat (like butter and cheese) is usually solid at room temperature, and unsaturated fat (like cooking oils) is liquid.

3 Mozaffarian, D. (2016). Dietary and Policy Priorities for Cardiovascular Disease, Diabetes, and Obesity – A Comprehensive Review. *Circulation*, 133(2), 187-225.

4 Estruch, R., Ros, E., Salas-Salvadó, J., Covas, M.I., Corella, D., Arós, F., Gómez-Gracia, E., Ruiz-Gutiérrez, V., Fiol, M., Lapetra, J., Lamuela-Raventos, R.M., Serra-Majem, L., Pintó, X., Basora, J., Muñoz, M.A., Sorlí, J.V., Martínez, J.A., Fitó, M., Gea, A., Hernán, M.A., & Martínez-González, M.A. (2018). Primary Prevention of Cardiovascular Disease with a Mediterranean Diet Supplemented with Extra-Virgin Olive Oil or Nuts. *New England Journal of Medicine*, 378(25).

Lignans are one of the major polyphenols in extra virgin olive oil, and are notably absent from its culinary competitors, such as oils made from seeds.

Another olive oil phenol, hydroxytyrosol, has the rare status of having a specific health benefit recognised by the European Food Safety Authority. The Authority accepted in 2011 that hydroxytyrosol stops oxidation of cholesterol, a key step in atherosclerosis (see Keeping the lines open). The official recognition read:[5]

> On the basis of the data presented, the Panel concludes that a cause and effect relationship has been established between the consumption of olive oil polyphenols (standardised by the content of hydroxytyrosol and its derivatives) and protection of LDL [cholesterol] particles from oxidative damage.

Hydroxytyrosol is the only phenol based molecule, from any source, to bear this honour.

There is also credible evidence oleocanthal and another major olive oil polyphenol called oleuropein (hydroxytyrosol comes from breaking up oleuropein), fend off dementia, at least in part by antagonising inflammation. In fact oleuropein has multiple antioxidant and anti-inflammatory properties, and evidence, at least at the level of cells grown in laboratories, of mitigating numerous types of cancer.

Quality is vital. The healthiest oils, with the most polyphenols, are the sharpest and greenest, and the difference lies in the making. Olive oil no longer comes from a stone mill turned by a melancholic donkey. At its best, olives are mashed with water and spun in a centrifuge; at its more dubious, they are hammered with cooking[6] and solvents, so read the label. *Virgin* and *extra virgin* are regulated terms for the richest and least damaged oil; *refined* and simply *olive oil* are more basic.

---

5   EFSA Panel on NDA , (2011). Polyphenols in olive related health claims. *EFSA Journal*, 9(4), 2033.
6   The warning applies to other cooking oils as well; heat treatment is often used to extract oil from plant material, and destroys a lot of the natural goodness.

Polyphenols explain why olive oil is useable long after you open it. Oil is spoiled by oxygen, the same way your tissues are (free radicals are oxygen – see The inflammage), and polyphenols stop it happening. In fact, polyphenols permeate every part of an olive tree (which is intriguing seeing it survives centuries in dust and hot sun), and recent interest has turned to their leaves. Olive leaves were once no more use than a folk remedy; infused in hot water they treated fevers like malaria. But most orchard prunings were put on a bonfire, or fed to goats. We now know that the leaves of an olive tree have exceptional antioxidants with even more anti-inflammatory polyphenols (mainly oleuropein) than the oil. One review found 1,450 milligrams of phenols in 100 grams of leaves, but only 110 of them in the same weight of fruit, and 23 in 100 millilitres of oil.[7]

Olive leaf extracts block various steps in the inflammation pathway and scavenge the free radicals which are a major cause of age-related inflammation. They have several times the free radical scavenging power of vitamin C and green tea, and reduce oxidative stress in the organs of aged rats.[8] They suppress inflammatory atherosclerosis in rabbits.[9] Information from humans is limited, but some studies show that in addition to their anti-inflammatory properties, olive leaf extracts lower blood pressure and improve circulating fat levels. The health industry has noticed them in the last decade or two, and commercial forces have mobilised to get them into the diet of health-

---

7   Lockyer, S., Rowland, I., Spencer, J., Yaqoob, P., & Stonehouse, W. (2016). Impact of phenolic-rich olive leaf extract on blood pressure, plasma lipids and inflammatory markers: a randomised controlled trial. *European Journal of Nutrition*, 56(4), 1421-1432.

8   Çoban, J., Öztezcan, S., Doğru-Abbasoğlu, S., Bingül, I., Yeşil-Mizrak, K., & Uysal, M. (2014). Olive leaf extract decreases age-induced oxidative stress in major organs of aged rats. *Geriatrics & Gerontology International*, 14(4), 996-1002.

9   Wang, L., Geng, C., Jiang, L. et al. (2008). The anti-atherosclerotic effect of olive leaf extract is related to suppressed inflammatory response in rabbits with experimental atherosclerosis. *European Journal of Nutrition*, 47, 235.

conscious people. Olive leaves and their extracts are marketed as tea, dietary supplements and leaf-enriched oil, and may prove to be the best the olive tree has to offer.

References
Aparicio-Soto, M., Sánchez-Hidalgo, M., Rosillo, M., Castejón, M., & Alarcón-de-la-Lastra, C. (2016). Extra virgin olive oil: a key functional food for prevention of immune-inflammatory diseases. *Food & Function,* 7(11), 4492-4505.

Aseem, M. (2013). Saturated fat is not the major issue. *BMJ,* 347:f6340.

Azaizeh, H., Halahlih, F., Najami, N., Brunner, D., Faulstich, M., & Tafesh, A. (2012). Antioxidant activity of phenolic fractions in olive mill wastewater. *Food Chemistry,* 134(4), 2226-2234.

Barbaro B, Toietta G, Maggio R, et al. (2014). Effects of the Olive-Derived Polyphenol Oleuropein on Human Health. Antonio S-C, ed. *International Journal of Molecular Sciences,* 15(10),18508-18524.

Bernardini, E., & Visioli, F. (2017). High quality, good health: The case for olive oil. *European Journal of Lipid Science and Technology,* 119(1).

Beauchamp, G.K., Russell, N., Keast, S.J., Morel, D., Lin, J., Pika, J., Han, Q., Lee, C-H., Smith, A.B., & Paul, A.S. (2005). Breslin Ibuprofen-like activity in extra-virgin olive oil. *Nature,* 437, 45–46.

Çoban, J., Öztezcan, S., Doğru-Abbasoğlu, S., Bingül, I., Yeşil-Mizrak, K., & Uysal, M. (2014). Olive leaf extract decreases age-induced oxidative stress in major organs of aged rats. *Geriatrics & Gerontology International,* 14(4), 996-1002.

Covas, M. (2008). Bioactive effects of olive oil phenolic compounds in humans: reduction of heart disease factors and oxidative damage. *Inflammopharmacology,* 16(5), 216-218.

Dieter, B., & Tuttle, K. (2017). Dietary strategies for cardiovascular health. *Trends in Cardiovascular Medicine,* 27(5), 295-313.

EFSA Panel on NDA , (2011). Polyphenols in olive related health claims. *EFSA Journal,* 9(4), 2033.

Estruch, R., Ro,s E., Salas-Salvadó, J., Covas, M.I., et al. (2013). Primary prevention of cardiovascular disease with a Mediterranean diet. *New England Journal of Medicine,* 368(14), 1279-90.

Lindsay, D., & Clifford, M. (2000). Oleuropein and related compounds. *Journal of the Science of Food and Agriculture,* 80(7), 1013-1023.

Lockyer, S., Rowland, I., Spencer, J., Yaqoob, P., & Stonehouse, W. (2016). Impact of phenolic-rich olive leaf extract on blood pressure, plasma lipids and inflammatory markers: a randomised controlled trial. *European Journal of Nutrition,* 56(4), 1421-1432.

Martín Peláez, S., Covas, M., Fitó, M., Kušar, A., & Pravst, I. (2013). Health effects of olive oil polyphenols: Recent advances and possibilities for the use of health claims. *Molecular Nutrition & Food Research,* 57(5), 760-771.

Mozaffarian, D. (2016). Dietary and Policy Priorities for Cardiovascular Disease, Diabetes, and Obesity – A Comprehensive Review. *Circulation,* 133(2), 187-225.

Omar, S. (2010). Oleuropein in Olive and its Pharmacological Effects. *Scientia Pharmaceutica,* 78(2), 133-154.

Owen, R., Mier, W., Giacosa, A., Hull, W., Spiegelhalder, B., & Bartsch, H. (2000). Identification of Lignans as Major Components in the Phenolic Fraction of Olive Oil. *Clinical Chemistry,* 46(7), 976.

Owen, R.W., Mier, W., Giacosa, A., Hul,l W.E., Spiegelhalder, B., & Bartsch, H. (2000). Phenolic compounds and squalene in olive oils: the concentration and antioxidant potential of total phenols, simple phenols, secoiridoids, lignans and squalene. *Food Chemistry Toxicology,* 38(8), 647-59.

Özcan, M., & Matthäus, B. (2016). A review: benefit and bioactive properties of olive (Olea europaea L.) leaves. *European Food Research and Technology,* 243(1), 89-99.

Pelletier, A., Barul, C., Féart, C., Helmer, C., Bernard, C., Periot, O., Dilharreguy, B., Dartigues, J., Allard, M., Barberger-Gateau, P., Catheline, G., & Samieri, C. (2015). Mediterranean diet and preserved brain structural connectivity in older subjects. *Alzheimer's and Dementia,* 11(9), 1023-1031.

Pérez Jiménez, F. (2007). Olive oil and oxidative stress. *Molecular Nutrition & Food Research,* 51(10), 1215-1224.

Pitt, J., Roth, W., Lacor, P., Smith, A., Blankenship, M., Velasco, P., De Felice, F., Breslin, P., & Klein, W. (2009). Alzheimer's-associated Aβ oligomers show altered structure, immunoreactivity and synaptotoxicity with low doses of oleocanthal. *Toxicology and Applied Pharmacology,* 240(2), 189-197.

Rahmanian, N., Jafari, S., & Wani, T. (2015). Bioactive profile, dehydration, extraction and application of the bioactive components of olive leaves. *Trends in Food Science & Technology,* 42(2), 150-172.

Reboredo-Rodriguez, P., Varela-Lopez, L., & Forbes-Hernandez, T.Y. (2018). Phenolic Compounds Isolated from Olive Oil as Nutraceutical Tools for the Prevention and Management of Cancer and Cardiovascular Diseases. *International Journal of Molecular Sciences,* 19(8), 2305.

Rigacci, S.(2015). Olive Oil Phenols as Promising Multi-targeting Agents Against Alzheimer's Disease. *Advances in Experimental Medicine and Biology,* 863, 1-20.

Scotece, M., Conde, J., Abella, V., Lopez, V., Pino, J., Lago, F., Smith, A., Gómez-Reino, J., & Gualillo, O. (2015). New drugs from ancient natural foods. Oleocanthal, the natural occurring spicy compound of olive oil: a brief history. *Drug Discovery Today,* 20(4), 406-410.

Singh, B., Parsaik, A., Mielke, M., Erwin, P., Knopman, D., Petersen, R., & Roberts, R. (2014). Association of Mediterranean Diet with Mild Cognitive Impairment and Alzheimer's Disease: A Systematic Review and Meta-Analysis. *Journal of Alzheimer's Disease,* 39(2), 271-282.

Souilem, S., Fki, I., Kobayashi, I., Khalid, N., Neves, M., Isoda, H., Sayadi, S., & Nakajima, M. (2016). Emerging Technologies for Recovery of Value-Added Components from Olive Leaves and Their Applications in Food/Feed Industries. *Food and Bioprocess Technology,* 10(2), 229-248.

Tresserra-Rimbau, A., Rimm, E., Medina-Remón, A., Martínez-González, M., López-Sabater, M., Covas, M., Corella, D., Jordi, S., Gómez-Gracia, E., Lapetra, J., Arós, F., Fiol, M., Ros, E., Serra-Majem, L., Xavier, P., Muñoz, M., Gea, A., Ruiz-Gutiérrez, V., Estruch, R., & Lamuela-Raventós, R. (2014). Polyphenol intake and mortality risk: a re-analysis of the PREDIMED trial. *BMC Medicine,* 12, 77-77.

Velasco, J., & Dobarganes, C. (2002). Oxidative stability of virgin olive oil. *European Journal of Lipid Science and Technology,* 104(9-10), 661-676.

Wang, L., Geng, C., Jiang, L. et al. (2008). The anti-atherosclerotic effect of olive leaf extract is related to suppressed inflammatory response in rabbits with experimental atherosclerosis. *European Journal of Nutrition,* 47, 235.

22

THE SECRET GARDEN

Get friendly with the right bacteria

We have long known that our bowels harbour bacteria which break down our food, particularly long-chain sugars (fibre), and make some of our vitamins (K for instance, and various forms of B). In return, we give them somewhere to live, and drop food on them. It is a successful arrangement. The average gut has 100 trillion of them, but they are far more than a compost heap. Bowel bugs have 100 times the genes of their human host, and a commensurate facility to make molecules that drive metabolism. New work ties their activities to outcomes as diverse as obesity, diabetes, blood pressure and psychiatric disease (they make the same chemicals, called neurotransmitters, the brain does). They also manipulate the immune system.

Your gut is a huge immune organ, because of its special status: it tolerates bugs normally repelled as invaders. Your bowel boundary keeps out all the noxious things you eat, and all the bacteria and fungi that work on it, but allows the molecules you need to filter in. It is quite a feat. Even useful bacteria would cause serious disease if they escaped, so nature has created a tolerant space inside a well-policed boundary. Intriguingly, to protect their niche, good bugs help maintain the fence. Some elegant experiments show the right bowel bugs make the joins between gut-lining epithelial cells tighter and more robust.

The implication is that strong joins depend on the type of bugs that butt up against them. At least some of the effect appears to arise from short-chain fatty acids, like butyrate, which bacteria in the large bowel make by fermenting starch. The crucial gut-lining cells use butyrate and its fellow travellers for food, and do better with a regular supply. When electric resistance is measured across layers of epithelial cells in a laboratory dish (an accepted approximation of permeability), the right fatty acids increase it.[1]

Bowel breaches matter because the wrong things in your bloodstream bring down the wrath of the immune system. Bacterial lipopolysaccharides, for instance, are large fat-cum-sugar molecules from bacterial cell walls, and they are found throughout the large bowel. They are also the prime signals the immune system relies on to notice when bacteria turn up somewhere dangerous, like your blood. So anticipate trouble when the bowel wall breaches and stray lipopolysaccharides squeeze through. As you get older, the bug balance in your gut tilts away from the ones that make the wall tight and it gets leakier. More and more of the wrong things filter out. There is plausible evidence this is a significant factor behind the inflammage. One intriguing strand of evidence comes from studies of centenarians' bowel complement which show their bacteria are often age-atypical.[2] Cause or effect? It would be nice to know.

Short-chain fatty acids appear capable of talking to tissues well beyond the gut, such as the liver, and dampening inflammation around joints. The field is new and growing, but microbiota-derived, short-chain fatty acids may well prove to be key mediators of cell functions

1   Cox, A.J., West, N.P., & Cripps, A.W. (2015). Obesity, inflammation, and the gut microbiota. *Lancet Diabetes Endocrinology*, 3.
2   Maffei, V., Kim, S., Blanchard, E., Luo, M., Jazwinski, S., Taylor, C., & Welsh, D. (2017). Biological Aging and the Human Gut Microbiota. *The Journals of Gerontology Series A: Biomedical Sciences and Medical Sciences*, 72(11), 1474-1482.

all over the body, possibly even the substantive link between diet, internal bacteria and health.

By chopping up big molecules so they can cross the gut wall, bacteria manage the food energy you absorb. When bowel bugs are transplanted from fat mice to thin ones, the thin ones get obese.[3] In other words, the tendency to get fat moves with the bugs. Obesity is a major stimulus of inflammation (see The fire in the fat), so harbouring bacteria that are sluggish at the splitting job is a good start towards avoiding it. Work is underway to see if transplanting the right bacteria could help people lose weight.

But there is more. Bacteria modulate satiety signals, which come from hormones that tell you when you have eaten enough. They also do good work chewing up the anti-inflammatory polyphenols you eat, which have to be liberated from molecules they were bound to before they become active.

So how can these insights be used? Bacteria come in manifold strains and species; good health requires the right ones, but it also requires diversity. A rainforest, not a pine plantation. Like everything alive, bacteria depend on their environment and, since they eat the same food you do, you have control. A rich array of fibrous plants gives you diverse and healthy bacteria, and a fat-ridden, low-fibre intake gives you limited ones. Bowel bugs, as in bad ones, may explain some of the way obesity and poor health follow in the wake of Western-style eating. But if your diet runs on well-known sensible lines – lots of diverse coloured plants – the bugs will follow. They are not a separate issue. They are another element of the good health payoff from eating properly. Likewise, calorie restriction, eating no more than you need, gives you good bugs and tight joins.

---

3   Martin, C.R., Osadchiy, V., Kalani, A., & Mayer, E.A. (2018). The Brain-Gut-Microbiome Axis. *Cellular and Molecular Gastroenterology and Hepatology*, 6(2), 133-148.

Work is in its infancy to see if major nutrition debates – like the role of meat and how many calories should come from grain – could be advanced by analysing the bowel flora of people on different diets.[4] In other words, which options promote the bacteria known to be healthy? Already personal variability has emerged as a significant factor. Experts speculate that when the data gets better, the day might dawn when health-aware people could have personal eating plans drawn up from the bugs the laboratory finds in their bowels.

Probiotics are cultures of bacteria in pills or food like yoghurt that, in theory, seed your gut when you eat them. Whether the complex ecosystem involved really responds in a lasting way to such treatment is uncertain. The evidence is inconclusive, and the argument that flora blooms when conditions (which means food) are right is powerful. Nobody plants rainforests.

Antibiotics disturb the normal arrangement and even short courses can disrupt things for years—a good argument for not taking them casually. Likewise, a healthy garden does not like the synthetic chemicals that arise in a lot of modern food, such as sweeteners and emulsifiers.

Tantalisingly, bacteria may explain some of the health benefits of nutraceuticals. Curcumin increases bacterial richness in the guts of mice.[5] Similar results in laboratory settings have been found with catechin (from tea), omega-3 fatty acids and grape seeds. In fact, several dozen plant polyphenols, including ones from major bioactive players like soy beans and berry fruit, appear to have this sort of influence.[6]

4   Milani, C., Ferrario, C., Turroni, F., Duranti, S., Mangifesta, M., Sinderen, D., & Ventura, M. (2016). The human gut microbiota and its interactive connections to diet. *Journal of Human Nutrition & Dietetics*, 29(5), 539-546.
5   Dudek-Wicher, R.K., Junka, A., & Bartoszewicz, M. (2018). The influence of antibiotics and dietary components on gut microbiota. *Przeglad Gastroenterologiczny*, 13(2), 85-92.
6   Carrera-Quintanar, L., López Roa, R.I., Quintero-Fabián, S., Sánchez-Sánchez, M.A., Vizmanos, B., & Ortuño-Sahagún, D. (2018). Phytochemicals That Influence Gut Microbiota as Prophylactics and for the Treatment of Obesity and Inflammatory Diseases. *Mediators of Inflammation*.

Although a grasp of the details remains on the distant horizon, the possibility is more than plausible that part of the anti-inflammatory magic of nutraceuticals arises from appealing to the right bacteria.

References
Azad, M.A.K., Sarker, M., Li, T., & Yin, J. (2018). Probiotic Species in the Modulation of Gut Microbiota: An Overview. *BioMed Research International*.

Belkaid, Y., & Hand, T.W. (2014). Role of the microbiota in immunity and inflammation. *Cell*, 157(1), 121-41.

Carrera-Quintanar, L., López Roa, R.I., Quintero-Fabián, S., Sánchez-Sánchez, M.A., Vizmanos, B., & Ortuño-Sahagún, D. (2018). Phytochemicals That Influence Gut Microbiota as Prophylactics and for the Treatment of Obesity and Inflammatory Diseases. *Mediators of Inflammation*.

Chung, H-J., Nguyen, T.T.B., Kim, H-J., & Hong, S-T. (2018). Gut Microbiota as a Missing Link Between Nutrients and Traits of Human. *Frontiers in Microbiology*, 9, 1510.

Cox, A.J., West, N.P.,& Cripps, A.W. (2015). Obesity, inflammation, and the gut microbiota. *Lancet Diabetes Endocrinology*, 3.

Dudek-Wicher, R.K., Junka, A., & Bartoszewicz, M. (2018). The influence of antibiotics and dietary components on gut microbiota. *Przeglad Gastroenterologiczny*, 13(2), 85-92.

Ferrucci, L., & Fabbri, E. (2018). Inflammageing: chronic inflammation in ageing, cardiovascular disease, and frailty. *Nature Reviews Cardiology*, 15(9), 505-522.

Jandhyala, S.M., Talukdar, R., Subramanyam, C., Vuyyuru, H., Sasikala, M., & Reddy, D.N. (2015). Role of the normal gut microbiota. *World Journal of Gastroenterology: WJG*, 21(29), 8787-8803.

Jiang, C., Li, G., Huang, P., Liu, Z., & Zhao, B. (2017). The Gut Microbiota and Alzheimer's Disease. *Journal of Alzheimer's Disease*, 58(1), 1-15.

Kang, Y., & Cai, Y. (2017). Gut microbiota and obesity: implications for fecal microbiota transplantation therapy. *Hormones*, 16(3), 223-234.

Kayshap, P., & Quigley, E. (2018). Therapeutic implications of the gastrointestinal microbiome. *Current Opinion in Pharmacology*, 38, 90-96.

Komaroff, A. (2018). The Microbiome and Risk for Atherosclerosis. *JAMA*, 319(23), 2381-2382.

Liu, L., & Zhu, G. (2018). Gut–Brain Axis and Mood Disorder. *Frontiers in Psychiatry*, 9, 223.

Maffei, V., Kim, S., Blanchard, E., Luo, M., Jazwinski, S., Taylor, C., & Welsh, D. (2017). Biological Aging and the Human Gut Microbiota. *The Journals of Gerontology Series A: Biomedical Sciences and Medical Sciences*, 72(11), 1474-1482.

Marques, C., Fernandes, I., Meireles, M., et al. (2018). Gut microbiota modulation accounts for the neuroprotective properties of anthocyanins. *Scientific Reports*, 8, 11341.

Martin, C.R., Osadchiy, V., Kalani, A., & Mayer, E.A. (2018). The Brain-Gut-Microbiome Axis. *Cellular and Molecular Gastroenterology and Hepatology*, 6(2), 133-148.

Meulen, T., Harmsen, H., Bootsma, H., Spijkervet, F., Kroese, F., & Vissink, A. (2016). The microbiome–systemic diseases connection. *Oral Diseases*, 22(8), 719-734.

Milani, C., Ferrario, C., Turroni, F., Duranti, S., Mangifesta, M., Sinderen, D., & Ventura, M. (2016). The human gut microbiota and its interactive connections to diet. *Journal of Human Nutrition & Dietetics*, 29(5), 539-546.

Rathinam, V., & Fitzgerald, K. (2013). Immunology Lipopolysaccharide sensing on the inside. *Nature*, 501(7466), 173-175.

Sonnenburg, J., & Bäckhed, F. (2016). Diet–microbiota interactions as moderators of human metabolism. *Nature*, 535(7610), 56-64.

Tengeler, A., Kozicz, T., & Kiliaan, A. (2018). Relationship between diet, the gut microbiota, and brain function. *Nutrition Reviews, Advance Article* (8), 1-617.

23

THE MANY-SEEDED APPLE
The ancient pomegranate

When hand-thrown explosives first became a viable force in armed combat, the inventors were struck, like all concept developers, with the need for a name. Word historians note the label they chose first appeared in the late sixteenth century and compared a hand-sized explosive to a fruit with hundreds of seeds. Grenades, therefore, are named for pomegranates, via Middle Ages French. And of all the historical influence this very ancient fruit has had, which is considerable, lending its name to a bomb is the most bizarre.

Pomegranates crop up in everything from medieval paintings of the Virgin Mary to Armenian wedding ceremonies (where the bride throws one against a wall), and Greek myth where Hades, god of the underworld, used one to stake his claim to the daughter of Zeus (fertility is something of a recurring theme). All the major religions attach symbolism to it, and ancient medicine linked it with numerous therapeutic properties. Archaeologists say people were eating pomegranate in various very early periods, such as Egypt and Mesopotamia, which puts it up there with the birth of civilisation. Modern research suggests they were wise to do so.

Cut open a pomegranate and hundreds of translucent red beads spill out. The beads are called arils, and each one contains a white seed (the name pomegranate means 'apple with many seeds'). Pomegranate has a slate of anti-inflammatory effects, and demonstrable benefit in warding off dementia, heart disease (atherosclerosis) and cancer. And every bit of the fruit counts: arils, pith and skin.

Pomegranates have more antioxidants than red wine or green tea.[1] Even the flowers are in on the act. Pomegranate flowers beat tea and wine by a factor of three. Pomegranates have only been on the nutraceutical radar since early this century, which is surprising, as they are one of the best examples of the concept and widely recommended by opinion leaders in the nutraceutical world.

Pomegranates are loaded with numerous desirable polyphenols, such as quercetin, catechin (also found in tea), and anthocyanins (that make them red). But the dominant class is tannins (ellagitannins and gallotannins) which often come through in high concentrations in the juice. Ellagitannins are large molecules which break down in the gut to small ones that are easily absorbed; they appear to carry the main thrust of the health effects.

One of pomegranate's most intriguing targets is the brain. When older people with mild memory impairment drink daily pomegranate juice they perform better on memory tests than matched companions who drink a placebo.[2] If rats are given the anti-anxiety drug Valium they lose the ability to perform memory tests such as mazes, but if they are dosed at the same time with extracts from pomegranate, the deficiency is reversed.[3]

1   Zarfeshany, A., Asgary, S., & Javanmard, S.H. (2014). Potent health effects of pomegranate. *Advanced Biomedical Research*, 3, 100.
2   Bookheimer, S.Y., et al. (2013). Pomegranate Juice Augments Memory and fMRI Activity in Middle-Aged and Older Adults with Mild Memory Complaints. *Evidence-based Complementary and Alternative Medicine : eCAM, PMC*.
3   Mansouri, M.T., Farbood, Y., Naghizadeh, B., Shabani, S., Mirshekar, M.A., & Sarkaki, A. (2016). Beneficial effects of ellagic acid against animal models of scopolamine- and diazepam-induced cognitive impairments. *Pharmaceutical Biology*, 1, 1-7.

Multiple sclerosis comes from slow patchy loss of a sheath called myelin that wraps around nerve cells like insulation on electric wire. Without myelin the nerve doesn't work. Mice don't get multiple sclerosis, so researchers cause something similar by injecting them with proteins that cause brain inflammation.[4] Researchers in Israel have shown that oil from pomegranate seeds dramatically (their word) reduced demyelination when fed to mice with inflamed demyelinating brains.[5]

It is well known that people can have memory difficulty after heart surgery. It probably occurs because cutting up the heart, putting clamps on the great vessels, and all the other clever manipulations that heart surgeons perform, throws off showers of tiny clots which float up to the brain. These clots cause damage in various ways, including oxidative stress. So can pomegranate help? Apparently it can. In one study in California, subjects who took a daily pomegranate extract before their heart operation, and continued for six weeks afterwards, did better in memory tests than age-matched patients who did not.[6]

It even helps when brains are permanently injured. Most of the brain's blood comes via the carotid arteries, and cutting them off leaves the brain pretty compromised. When this is done to rats, their ability to navigate mazes and other tests of their cognition is partially preserved if they eat pomegranate extract.[7]

A group of people with established heart disease (not healthy people trying to avoid it) were given pomegranate juice to drink

---

4 Called *experimental autoimmune encephalomyelitis*.
5 Binyamin, O., Larush, L., Frid, K., et al. (2015). Treatment of a multiple sclerosis animal model by a novel nanodrop formulation of a natural antioxidant. *International Journal of Nanomedicine*, 10, 7165-7174.
6 Ropacki, S.A., Patel, S.M., & Hartman, R.E. (2013). Pomegranate Supplementation Protects against Memory Dysfunction after Heart Surgery: A Pilot Study. *Evidence-Based Complementary and Alternative Medicine*.
7 Hajipour, S., Sarkaki, A., Mohammad, S., Mansouri, T., Pilevarian, A., & RafieiRad, M. (2014). Motor and cognitive defects due to permanent cerebral hypoperfusion/ischemia improve by pomegranate seed extract in rats. *Journal of Biological Sciences*, 17(8), 991-8.

daily. Another group were given something that looked and tasted the same. After three months, the pomegranate group had a statistically significant improvement in blood flow through their coronary arteries when they exercised.[8]

Pomegranate is also a major player in cancer prevention. Laboratory work on cultured cells imply it can play a role in preventing cancers of the skin, breast, prostate and bowel, which are some of the biggest cancers going.

It also seems to help fend off obesity, and some of obesity's complications, like diabetes and fatty liver. In one study pomegranate peel fed to laboratory animals on a high fat diet counteracted the fat-induced expression of inflammatory markers in both their guts and their fat tissue. The peel also promoted healthy gut bacteria. The researchers, from the Louvain Drug Research Institute in Belgium, concluded that '…pomegranate constitutes a promising food in the control of atherogenic and inflammatory disorders associated with diet-induced obesity.'[9]

As to getting hold of it, one option is to grow some. The trees do well in most environments, and are popular as ornamental shrubs, although you are unlikely to get enough for a daily dose. Whether home-grown or bought from the fruit shop, the arils are a versatile ingredient that go well in smoothies and as sprinkles on salads and cereals.

However, the easiest way to consume pomegranate every day is via juice or powder, which are arguably improvements on arils because they include the rich but inedible skin. The downside is the processing.

8   Sumner, M.D., Elliott-Eller, M., Weidner, G., Daubenmier, J.J., Chew, M.H., Marlin, R., Raisin, C.J., & Ornish, D. (2005). Effects of pomegranate juice consumption on myocardial perfusion in patients with coronary heart disease *American Journal of Cardiology*, 96(6), 810-4.
9   Neyrinck, A.M., Van Hée, V.F., Bindels, L.B., De Backer, F., Cani, P.D., & Delzenne, N.M. (2013). Polyphenol-rich extract of pomegranate peel alleviates tissue inflammation and hypercholestrolaemia in high-fat diet induced obese mice: potential implication of the gut microbiota. *British Journal of Nutrition*, 109(5), 802-9.

Phenols are cloudy and bitter, so even the best not-from-concentrate, no-additives juice is commonly filtered or dosed with enzymes, which kills a lot of the goodness. Processing can remove more than half the polyphenols the untreated juice held, according to some experiments. Even so, the polyphenols in a measure of processed juice every day will accumulate, and a daily shot is likely to be the most reliable practice over time.

References
http://www.etymonline.com/index.php?term=grenade

Al-Muammar, M., & Khan, F. (2012). Obesity: The preventive role of the pomegranate (Punica granatum). *Nutrition,* 28(6), 595-604.

Binyamin, O., Larush, L., Frid, K., et al. (2015). Treatment of a multiple sclerosis animal model by a novel nanodrop formulation of a natural antioxidant. *International Journal of Nanomedicine,* 10, 7165-7174.

Bookheimer, S.Y., et al. (2013). Pomegranate Juice Augments Memory and fMRI Activity in Middle-Aged and Older Adults with Mild Memory Complaints. *Evidence-based Complementary and Alternative Medicine : eCAM, PMC.*

Farahmand, M., Golmakani, M., Mesbahi, G., & Farahnaky, A. (2017). Investigating the Effects of Large-Scale Processing on Phytochemicals and Antioxidant Activity of Pomegranate Juice. *Journal of Food Processing and Preservation,* 41(2).

Fischer, U., Dettmann, J., Carle, R., & Kammerer, D. (2011). Impact of processing and storage on the phenolic profiles and contents of pomegranate (Punica granatum L.) juices. *European Food Research and Technology,* 233(5), 797-816.

Hajipour, S., Sarkaki, A., Mohammad, S., Mansouri, T., Pilevarian, A.,& RafieiRad, M. (2014). Motor and cognitive defects due to permanent cerebral hypoperfusion/ischemia improve by pomegranate seed extract in rats. *Journal of Biological Sciences,* 17(8), 991-8.

Horwitz, S. (2006). The Power of the Pomegranate: Biblical Fruit with Medicinal Properties. *Alternative and Complementary Therapies,* 121-126.

Kang, I., Buckner, T., Shay, N., Gu, L., & Chung, S. (2016). Improvements in Metabolic Health with Consumption of Ellagic Acid and Subsequent Conversion into Urolithins: Evidence and Mechanisms. *Advances in Nutrition,* 7(5), 961-972.

Mansouri, M.T., Farbood, Y., Naghizadeh, B., Shabani, S., Mirshekar, M.A., & Sarkaki, A. (2016). Beneficial effects of ellagic acid against animal models of scopolamine- and diazepam-induced cognitive impairments. *Pharmaceutical Biology,* 1, 1-7.

Medjakovic, S., & Jungbauer, A. (2012). Pomegranate: a fruit that ameliorates metabolic syndrome. *Food & Function,* 4(1), 19-39.

Mirsaeedghazi, H., Emam-Djomeh, Z., Mousavi, S., Aroujalian, A., & Navidbakhsh, M. (2010). Clarification of pomegranate juice by microfiltration with PVDF membranes. *Desalination,* 264(3), 243-248.

Ropacki, S.A., Patel, S.M., & Hartman, R.E. (2013). Pomegranate Supplementation Protects against Memory Dysfunction after Heart Surgery: A Pilot Study. *Evidence Based Complementary Alternative Medicine.*

Ruis, A. (2015). Pomegranate and the Mediation of Balance in Early Medicine. Gastronomica: *The Journal of Food and Culture,* 15(1).

Sharma, P., McClees, S.F., & Afaq, F. (2017). Pomegranate for Prevention and Treatment of Cancer: An Update. *Molecules,* 22(1), E177.

Turrini, E., Ferruzzi, L., Fimognari, C. (2015). Potential Effects of Pomegranate Polyphenols in Cancer Prevention and Therapy. *Oxidative Medicine and Cellular Longevity.*

Zarfeshany, A., Asgary, S., & Javanmard, S.H. (2014). Potent health effects of pomegranate. *Advanced Biomedical Research,* 3, 100.

24

DEADLY WHITE POWDER
The seduction of sugar

The appeal of sweetness is deeply rooted in the human psyche and shows itself from the earliest years of life. It touches everybody, regardless of race or culture, and probably happens because fruit, the original dietary sweetness, was once rare and desirable. Sugar stimulates the same part of the brain as morphine, so the pleasure reward for eating it is considerable. Unfortunately, so are the consequences. We no longer collect the occasional handful of medieval blueberries, and the food industry, which knows very well what mesmerises consumers, saturate their offerings with it. We are now at the point where any food that didn't 'grow like that' is likely to have sugar added, including ones that are not obvious, like yoghurt, muesli and tomato sauce. In fact anything in a can, bottle or foil wrapper is at risk, even ostensibly wholesome options, so avoiding sugar is far more complicated than just avoiding confectionary.[1]

The food industry knows the problem, and puts out its own scientific literature. So the debate about where the health consequences fall,

---

1 Sugar balances sour and salty ingredients to create a composite taste that is not sweet. It also contributes texture or 'mouth feel', like fat. For these reasons even savoury food like soup, ready meals and canned vegetables often have added sugar. 'Fat-free' items are a particular trap; they rely on sugar to remain palatable in the absence of fat. Furthermore, the issue is often clouded by the plethora of terms, like glucose, dextrose, cane juice, malt syrup etc. that appear on ingredient labels in place of sugar.

especially when the evidence is incomplete and derivative (such as with animal studies), has a commercially tinged ferocity.

The principal problem is energy. Sweet food is energy dense, another reason premodern people gravitated towards it, and eating more than a little lays down fat. Excess fat is intensely inflammatory, as per The fire in the fat, and a major modern health issue. Sugary food is particularly adept at sticking fat around your organs and inside your liver, which is by far the most dangerous place for it.

Obesity has increased over the last forty years in a fairly close parallel to the amount of sugar added to food,[2] and there are calls from some quarters to tax sugar like alcohol and tobacco and restrict its sale.

Even so, energy is not the end of it. Sugar has implications for major conditions such as heart disease and cognitive impairment even when the effect of body weight is removed. At least some of the basis for this is inflammation. Separating out the effects of weight is difficult for human subjects, so the insights, which are intriguing, come largely from animals. So there is plenty of room for argument.

Two molecules, glucose and fructose, are key. For several hundred years the dominant added sweetener was sucrose, or table sugar, which comes from tropical sugar cane. Sucrose consists of a molecule each of glucose and fructose stuck together. For the last few decades industrial sweetness in some parts of the world has increasingly come from an ingredient called high-fructose corn syrup, used particularly in soft drinks. Despite its name, high-fructose corn syrup is also equal parts of glucose and fructose, which finds favour with the industrial world because it is cheap and easier to manipulate chemically than sucrose.

---

2   Malik, V., & Hu, F. (2015). Fructose and Cardiometabolic Health. *Journal of the American College of Cardiology*, 66(14), A1-A34.

When you eat sucrose or corn syrup, the glucose and fructose molecules are split up, and reach your blood stream separately. Undoubtedly too much glucose is an energy-excess problem, but glucose is also the common currency of good food. When you eat cabbage or carrots or indeed most things, a large part of it enters your blood stream as glucose. Your body recognises it and knows what to do. Every cell runs on it. Business as usual. Not so for its fellow traveller.

Before sugar cane, which became available only after America was discovered, people ate very little fructose. Fructose in its whole food state is principally the sugar of fruit, which used to be rare, and autumnal, and it often got no better for most people than the occasional quince or Royal Russet apple. Which, incidentally, were much tarter than the modern sugary cultivars. So fructose has a specialised job: it goes to fat. In particular, abdominal fat. That is because it came into the diet before winter, when energy was stored. Perfectly sensible, particularly when there wasn't much of it.

Today fructose in industrial food is consumed far beyond its status in the natural scheme of things. The machinery that stores fat at harvest time ticks over all year on white bread and bottled fizz; indeed, it ticks over all year on most things the supermarket sells.

Bear in mind, as per The fire in the fat, the most inflammatory fat, which is the fat in and around your organs, is a negligible proportion of body weight. It can be significant even in people who tip the scales at a healthy level. The issue is what you eat, not necessarily what you weigh, and appearing to get away with the wrong choices is false reassurance.

Fructose is inflammatory. Within one week of a high-fructose diet the heart and blood cells of laboratory rats put out excess reactive oxygen species which are major inflammatory stimuli.[3] Mice fed high-sugar diets

---

3 Delbosc, S., Paizanis, E., Magous, R., et al. (2005). Involvement of oxidative stress and NADPH oxidase activation in the development of cardiovascular complications in a model of insulin resistance, the fructose-fed rat. *Atherosclerosis*, 179(1), 43-49.

get inflamed livers from the fructose component, which excites various inflammatory factors, particularly the ubiquitous NF-κB.[4]

Several studies have associated fructose intake with infiltration of white blood cells into fat tissue.[5] Fructose also pushes up levels of the key cytokine leptin, which further aggravates inflammation and releases reactive oxygen species.

High-sugar diets impair various types of thinking such as spatial perception and memory, and affect all age groups: learning in children and university students, and age-related decline, even dementia, in older people. The effects can be shown in experiments after mere days of exposure so weight gain cannot be the cause. Running the experiments on laboratory rats shows the issue is inflammation in specific parts of the brain, such as the hippocampus, which is a key structure in forming memories.[6]

None of this should cause doubt about consuming sugar, including fructose, in non-processed food. It is improbable that deleterious effects could arise from eating fruit, the major source of fructose, even by eating it regularly. Fruit, particularly berries, are some of the richest sources of anti-inflammatory polyphenols, and consumption – within reason – is to be encouraged. If the world just ate sugar in the form it grew, as an apple or a raspberry, without the dead hand of food scientists and their paraphernalia of food corruption, the issue would fold its tent and slink away.

4 Charrez, B., Qiao, L., & Hebbard, L. (2015). The role of fructose in metabolism and cancer. *Hormone Molecular Biology and Clinical Investigation*, 22(2), 80.

5 DiNicolantonio, J., Mehta, V., Onkaramurthy, N., & O'Keefe, J. (2018). Fructose-induced inflammation and increased cortisol: A new mechanism for how sugar induces visceral adiposity. *Progress in Cardiovascular Diseases*, 61(1), 3-9.

6 Beilharz, J., Maniam, J., & Morris, M. (2016). Short-term exposure to a diet high in fat and sugar, or liquid sugar, selectively impairs hippocampal-dependent memory, with differential impacts on inflammation. *Behavioural Brain Research*, 306, 1-7.

References

Beilharz, J., Maniam, J., & Morris, M. (2016). Short-term exposure to a diet high in fat and sugar, or liquid sugar, selectively impairs hippocampal-dependent memory, with differential impacts on inflammation. *Behavioural Brain Research, 306,* 1-7.

Bray, G.A. (2007). How bad is fructose? *American Journal of Clinical Nutrition,* 86(4), 895-896.

Cantley, L. (2013). Cancer, metabolism, fructose, artificial sweeteners, and going cold turkey on sugar. *BMC Biology,* 12, 3.

Charrez, B., Qiao, L., & Hebbard, L. (2015). The role of fructose in metabolism and cancer. *Hormone Molecular Biology and Clinical Investigation,* 22(2), 80.

Chiavaroli, L., Ha, V., de Souza, R., Kendall, C., & Sievenpiper, J. (2014). Fructose in obesity and cognitive decline: is it the fructose or the excess energy? *Nutrition Journal,* 13, 27.

de Souza, R., Jenkins, D., & Sievenpiper, J. (2012). Sugar: fruit fructose is still healthy. *Nature,* 482(7386), 470-470.

Delbosc, S., Paizanis, E., Magous, R., et al. (2005). Involvement of oxidative stress and NADPH oxidase activation in the development of cardiovascular complications in a model of insulin resistance, the fructose-fed rat. *Atherosclerosis,* 179(1), 43-49.

DiNicolantonio, J., Lucan, S., & O'Keefe, J. (2016). The Evidence for Saturated Fat and for Sugar Related to Coronary Heart Disease. *Progress in Cardiovascular Diseases,* 58(5), 464-472.

DiNicolantonio, J., Mehta, V., Onkaramurthy, N., & O'Keefe, J. (2018). Fructose-induced inflammation and increased cortisol: A new mechanism for how sugar induces visceral adiposity. *Progress in Cardiovascular Diseases,* 61(1), 3-9

Ferder, L., Ferder, M., & Inserra, F. (2010). The Role of High-Fructose Corn Syrup in Metabolic Syndrome and Hypertension. *Current Hypertension Reports,* 12(2), 105-112.

Jiang, Y., Pan, Y., Rhea, P.R., et al. (2016). A Sucrose-Enriched Diet Promotes Tumorigenesis in Mammary Gland in Part through the 12-Lipoxygenase Pathway. *Cancer Research,* 76(1), 24-29.

Mennella, J., & Bobowski, N. (2015). The sweetness and bitterness of childhood: Insights from basic research on taste preferences. *Physiology & Behavior,* 152(B), 502–507.

Schmidt, L., Brindis, C., & Lustig, R. (2012). Public health. The toxic truth about sugar. *Nature,* 482(7383), 27-29.

Tappy, L., & Lê, K. (2010). Metabolic Effects of Fructose and the Worldwide Increase in Obesity. *Physiological Reviews,* 90(1), 23-39.

Weichselbaum, E. (2008). Fruit makes you fat? *Nutrition Bulletin,* 33(4). 345.

White, J., (2008). Straight talk about high-fructose corn syrup: what it is and what it ain't. *American Journal of Clinical Nutrition,* 88(6), 1716S-1721S.

25

I THINK THEREFORE I AM

How thoughts move molecules

When Shakespeare wrote 'there is nothing either good or bad but thinking makes it so',[1] he was talking about how we view the world. Whether he intended it or not (Shakespeare was good at multiple meanings), he could also have been talking about health. People have known for millennia that staying well has a lot to do with thinking. Long before scalpels and pill bottles had any influence, techniques that directed thoughts into healthy channels were highly developed, particularly in Asia, and they remain popular worldwide. Today we call it meditation, and there are thousands of variations. Thing is, it works.

Meditation, regardless of type, has many targets; it is not just about feeling happier, or curing addictions. Meditation changes your chemistry. There is evidence that it lowers blood pressure, reduces cholesterol, and reduces by impressive margins the risk of big diseases like cancer and heart attacks. It also has no downside other than time expended. Medical schools and university researchers routinely acknowledge it and it is recognised by major wellness players such as the American Heart Association.[2]

---

1 Hamlet Act 2 Scene 2.
2 Levine, G.N., Richard A. Lange, C. Noel Bairey-Merz, et al. (2017). Meditation and Cardiovascular Risk Reduction A Scientific Statement From the American Heart Association. *Journal of the American Heart Association*, 6(10).

One of the big benefits at the cutting edge of meditation insights, and an excellent illustration of how deep the mind body connection goes, is your immune system. The hard data remains tentative, and it does not all point in the same direction, but various studies show solid clues that meditation changes our cells and their molecular processes for the better, particularly in respect of inflammation and ageing.

Research into the blood cells of people who meditate has shown they secrete fewer cytokines and show less oxidative stress. For instance, one study of 96 people showed that only 12 weeks of yoga-type meditation reduced various measures of cell ageing such as oxidative stress, which is a potent stimulus of inflammation, and the blood markers of DNA damage.[3]

Meditation's payoff makes sense when seen as the reverse of stress. It has long been known that inflammatory blood markers are higher in people under sustained personal stress, such as those who look after disabled relatives. They are also higher in people on low incomes, and people who had difficult childhoods. Population studies show that health improves as status, income and work satisfaction do, particularly for big-ticket items like heart disease. The relative absence of grinding daily stress at the higher end of the social ladder is part of the reason. Various mechanisms contribute, but a core observation is that stress turns on the genes that make the proteins of the inflammation response.

As per Epigenetics, and food as information, adverse life events affect the way genes are read, particularly in immune cells. When people pass through one of life's low points such as bereavement, the inflammatory genes in their white blood cells are switched on.

---

3 Tolahunase, M., Sagar, R., & Dada, R. (2017). Impact of Yoga and Meditation on Cellular Aging in Apparently Healthy Individuals: A Prospective, Open-Label Single-Arm Exploratory Study. *Oxidative Medicine and Cellular Longevity*, 2017, 7928981.

There is even a new academic field called *social genomics* to study the phenomenon.

Trials have demonstrated that activation of pro-inflammatory genes can be reversed by well-known meditation systems like Tai Chi and yoga. A key point of influence is NF-κB, the protein that controls when inflammatory genes are read. Several studies, covering groups as diverse as the lonely elderly and women with breast cancer, show that people have less of it in their blood cells after they have meditated.[4]

Potentially the most exciting impact for ageing is on telomeres. DNA gets frayed at the ends when it replicates, which it does when a cell divides. After so many divisions, it is no longer useable and the cell dies; dead cells provoke an inflammatory clean-up, as described in The inflammage. The ends of DNA have caps called telomeres, and it is the fitness of telomeres that determines how fast the fraying occurs. Robust cells have long ones. Telomeres are a clock; they tell your biological age. If you are getting older faster than your years, the telomeres will record it.

A study in Spain matched 20 members of a Buddhist community who practised a Zen breathing meditation with another 20 people of like age and lifestyle; the meditators were heavier than the comparison group and exercised less, but still had dramatically longer telomeres.[5] Other studies have found similar results, including patients with prostate cancer, and those who had undergone radiation for cancer of the breast. Measurable changes in small groups followed for short periods of time imply that the outcome of sustained meditation could be impressive.

---

4   Black, D., & Slavich, G. (2016). Mindfulness meditation and the immune system: a systematic review of randomized controlled trials. *Annals of the New York Academy of Sciences*, 1373(1), 13-24.

5   Alda, M., Puebla-Guedea, M., Rodero, B., Demarzo, M., Montero-Marin, J., Roca, M., & Garcia-Campayo, J. (2016). Zen meditation, Length of Telomeres, and the Role of Experiential Avoidance and Compassion. *Mindfulness*, 7(3), 651-659.

Telomeres are protected by an enzyme called telomerase, and another way of getting a handle on a cell's telomere situation is to measure telomerase activity. In 2011, a study showed for the first time – and several subsequent studies have agreed – that a group of people who did a course of meditation had more active telomerase enzymes than a matched group who did not.[6]

Likewise DNA methylation. As per Epigenetics, and food as information, your DNA gets more methylation pins stuck in it as you get older; this stops it being read properly, and the extent of the pincushion in certain key sites is an age marker. If the clock is running faster than you are, a common outcome of stress, the chances of a major disease increase. A recent study comparing 18 people who had meditated for at least three years with 20 age and sex-matched people who had not, found that the epigenetic ageing rate in the meditators decreased significantly with the number of years they had done it.[7] The effect was most marked for the ones over 50, implying the benefit is cumulative.

Mindfulness meditation has been shown to influence some of the same mechanisms that anti-inflammatory pharmaceuticals act upon. In the words of one recent paper,[8]

> Chronic low-grade inflammation is associated with the most common health problems in the modern world including cardiovascular and metabolic disease, cancer and neuropsychiatric disorders. Our findings suggest that mindfulness-based behavioral interventions

6   Jacobs, T.L., Epel, E.S., Lin, J., Blackburn, E.H., et al. (2011). Intensive meditation training, immune cell telomerase activity, and psychological mediators. *Psychoneuroendocrinology*, 36(5), 664-81.

7   Chaix, R., Alvarez-López, M.J., Fagny, M., et al. (2017). Epigenetic clock analysis in long-term meditators. *Psychoneuroendocrinology*, 85, 210-214.

8   Kaliman, P., Álvarez-López, M.J., Cosín-Tomás, M., Rosenkranz, M.A., Lutz, A., & Davidson, R.J. (2014). Rapid changes in histone deacetylases and inflammatory gene expression in expert meditators. *Psychoneuroendocrinology*, 40, 96-107.

may produce beneficial effects in subjects with chronic diseases in whom inflammation is a significant correlate. Data presented here suggest that mindfulness meditation practice influences mechanisms similar to those targeted by different anti-inflammatory drugs...

So spare a thought for thinking. It calms more than your mind and your mood.

References

Alda, M., Puebla-Guedea, M., Rodero, B., Demarzo, M., Montero-Marin, J., Roca, M., & Garcia-Campayo, J. (2016). Zen meditation, Length of Telomeres, and the Role of Experiential Avoidance and Compassion. *Mindfulness*, 7(3), 651-659.

Black, D., & Slavich, G. (2016). Mindfulness meditation and the immune system: a systematic review of randomized controlled trials. *Annals of the New York Academy of Sciences*, 1373(1), 13-24.

Bower, J.E., & Irwin, M.R. (2016). Mind-body therapies and control of inflammatory biology: A descriptive review. *Brain, Behavior, and Immunity*, 51, 1-11.

Chaix, R., Alvarez-López, M.J., Fagny, M., et al. (2017). Epigenetic clock analysis in long-term meditators. *Psychoneuroendocrinology*, 85, 210-214.

Deak, T., Kudinova, A., Lovelock, D.F., Gibb, B.E., & Hennessy, M.B. (2017). A multispecies approach for understanding neuroimmune mechanisms of stress. *Dialogues in Clinical Neuroscience*, 19(1), 37-53.

Deng, W., Cheung, S.T., Tsao, S.W., Wang, X.M., & Tiwari, A.F. (2016). Telomerase activity and its association with psychological stress, mental disorders, lifestyle factors and interventions: A systematic review. *Psychoneuroendocrinology*, 64, 150-63.

Epel, E., Daubenmier, J., Moskowitz, J.T., Folkman, S., & Blackburn, E. (2009). Can meditation slow rate of cellular aging? Cognitive stress, mindfulness, and telomeres. *Annals of the New York Academy of Sciences*, 1172, 34-53.

Fioranelli, M., Bottaccioli, A.G., Bottaccioli, F., Bianchi, M., Rovesti, M., & Roccia, M.G. (2018). Stress and Inflammation in Coronary Artery Disease: A Review Psychoneuroendocrineimmunology-Based. *Frontiers in Immunology*, 9, 2031.

Jacobs, T.L., Epel, E.S., Lin, J., Blackburn, E.H., et al. (2011). Intensive meditation training, immune cell telomerase activity, and psychological mediators. *Psychoneuroendocrinology*, 36(5), 664-81.

Kaliman, P., Álvarez-López, M.J., Cosín-Tomás, M., Rosenkranz, M.A., Lutz, A., & Davidson, R.J. (2014). Rapid changes in histone deacetylases and inflammatory gene expression in expert meditators. *Psychoneuroendocrinology*, 40, 96-107.

Koike, M., & Cardoso, R. (2014). Meditation can produce beneficial effects to prevent cardiovascular disease. *Hormone Molecular Biology and Clinical Investigation*, 18(3).

Kok, B., Waugh, C., & Fredrickson, B. (2013). Meditation and Health: The Search for Mechanisms of Action. *Social and Personality Psychology Compass,* 7(1).

Levine, G.N., Richard A. Lange, C. Noel Bairey-Merz, et al. (2017). Meditation and Cardiovascular Risk Reduction A Scientific Statement From the American Heart Association. *Journal of the American Heart Association,* 6(10).

Morgan, N., Irwin, M.R., Chung, M., & Wang, C. (2014). The Effects of Mind-Body Therapies on the Immune System: Meta-Analysis. *Bacurau RFP,* 9(7).

Rathore, M., & Abraham, J. (2018). Implication of Asana, Pranayama and Meditation on Telomere Stability. *International Journal of Yoga,* 11(3), 186-193.

Schutte, N.S., & Malouff, J.M. (2014). A meta-analytic review of the effects of mindfulness meditation on telomerase activity. *Psychoneuroendocrinology,* 42, 45-8.

Tolahunase, M., Sagar, R., & Dada, R. (2017). Impact of Yoga and Meditation on Cellular Aging in Apparently Healthy Individuals: A Prospective, Open-Label Single-Arm Exploratory Study. *Oxidative Medicine and Cellular Longevity,* 2017, 7928981.

26

WAKE UP AND SMELL...
The power of the morning cup

Somewhat surprisingly, the biggest sources of natural antioxidants in the average diet are not just fruit and vegetables. Although fruit and vegetables are the foundation of good eating, their contribution of dietary anti-inflammatory polyphenols is rivalled by tea and coffee.[1] The aroma that gets you out of bed, and the caffeine that makes your heart race, come from leaves and berries, along with thousands of other substances that massage your metabolism. Many of them are good for it, and multiple studies show moderate tea and coffee drinkers are better off in various ways for their daily habit.

Tea is rich in polyphenol flavonoids (see <u>Nutraceuticals and where they come from</u>), particularly a group called catechins. Polyphenols give tea bite and astringency and form anything up to thirty-five per cent of the weight of green leaves.[2] They also suppress various inflammatory diseases of the heart and brain, and some types of cancer.

Two grams of tea leaves, a standard tea bag, give up 150–200 mg of flavonoids when doused with hot water.[3] Most people consume no

1   Zamora-Ros, R., Rothwell, J.A., Scalbert, A., et al. (2013). Dietary intakes and food sources of phenolic acids in the European Prospective Investigation into Cancer and Nutrition (EPIC) study. *British Journal of Nutrition*, 110(8), 1500-11.
2   Dufresne, C., & Farnworth, E. (2000). Tea, Kombucha, and health: a review. *Food Research International*, 33(6), 409-421.
3   Hodgson, J., & Croft, K. (2010). Tea flavonoids and cardiovascular health. *Molecular Aspects of Medicine*, 31(6), 495-502.

more than 1,000 mg of flavonoids a day, and many quite a bit less, so the contribution of tea is considerable.

Coffee is also loaded with polyphenols, up to ten per cent of the weight of green beans, most of which are powerful antioxidants called chlorogenic acids. Although there is a lot of variation, an average cup contains several hundred milligrams of them, and regular coffee drinkers consume 1–2 grams a day, far exceeding any other source. A cup of coffee has more antioxidants than a glass of red wine.[4] People drinking coffee in lab conditions have more measurable antioxidant activity in their blood samples than comparable water drinkers, and population studies with thousands of subjects show people who drink coffee live longer.[5]

Coffee seems efficacious in warding off brain diseases like dementia and Parkinson's. The information is patchy, but drinking a few cups a day, not too many, seems to keep the brain ticking over, and a polyphenol called quercetin seems to be responsible.

Coffee also reduces the risk of liver cancer, and probably bowel cancer as well, although evidence for other cancers is mixed. Molecular studies show that various components of coffee inhibit the tiny new blood vessels that cancers make to feed themselves as well as the enzymes they use to break down surrounding tissue when they spread to new sites.

Various studies have indicated that coffee appears to reduce the risk of type 2 diabetes, the age-onset type, by anything up to sixty per cent.[6] It also reduces the risk of heart disease, which is the pathology most of us should worry about as we get older.

4   Yashin, A., Yashin, Y., Wang, J.Y., & Nemzer, B. (2013). Antioxidant and Antiradical Activity of Coffee. *Antioxidants*, 2(4), 230-245.
5   Ding, M., Satija, A., Bhupathiraju, S.N., et al. (2015). Association of Coffee Consumption with Total and Cause-Specific Mortality in Three Large Prospective Cohorts. *Circulation*, 132(24), 2305-2315.
6   Ludwig, I., Clifford, M., Lean, M., Ashihara, H., & Crozier, A. (2014). Coffee: biochemistry and potential impact on health. *Food & Function*, 5(8), 1695-1717.

This does not mean it is wrong for dietary advice to emphasise coloured plants ahead of espresso. Polyphenols are effective via their range, not just their quantity. It also doesn't mean these beverages, which both contain caffeine, should be consumed in excess, or that they are wholesome in any form. Both tea and coffee are commonly drunk with sugar, which is undesirable; coffee also attracts whipped cream and marshmallows, and is not a health drink when overloaded with them.

The antioxidant power of coffee's chlorogenic acids used to be undisputed. However, modern insights suggest they are of little use in mopping up free radicals on their own. Their effects on chronic inflammatory diseases are deeper and more complex. Although the data is not completely consistent, coffee drinkers have a lower risk of dying prematurely of an inflammatory disease, and the latest insights on how it works focus on gene expression (see Epigenetics, and food as information). Certain genes cause degenerative diseases by coding for proteins that form complex signalling cascades, and chlorogenic acids appear to work by blocking them. They are known to block NF-κB. Gene inhibition is particularly marked in the liver, which is a neat fit to studies that show coffee protects against cancer there, as well as cirrhosis and fatty liver deposits.

Tea takes dozens of forms – oolong, white, gunpowder, brick – depending on how it is treated, but two will do for discussion purposes: green and black. Green tea consists of the leaves straight off the bush, more or less, and black tea consists of leaves when dried and oxidised. Oxidation destroys some polyphenols, but makes new ones, and both forms of tea are rich in them. The oxidation of tea is called fermentation, which is something of a misnomer as it uses enzymes, not yeast, although some specialised teas really are fermented with microorganisms. Asian countries tend to drink green tea, and everywhere else tends to drink black. This means the subject tea in population studies comes down to where the research was conducted, but both types deliver substantial benefit.

Atherosclerotic plaques, the fatty deposits that cause heart attacks and strokes, grow more slowly in moderate, daily tea drinkers than in people who abstain. A study of half a million Chinese people recently reported a lower rate of heart disease in regular tea drinkers.[7] Another major piece of research combined the data from multiple other studies (known in the trade as a meta-analysis) and found that three cups of tea a day reduced the risk of a heart attack by eleven per cent.[8] Similar analysis has shown the same regime, three cups a day, reduces the risk of stroke.[9]

Another study in China of more than 7,000 'oldest old' people – those who are 80 years or more – found regular tea drinkers got better scores on thinking tests.[10] A similar investigation found the tea drinkers also lived longer.[11]

Both green and black tea inhibit cancer in mice, but studies on humans are mixed. Tea seems to suppress some cancers, such as skin and kidney, and have no effect on others, like breast.

Worldwide, only water is drunk in greater volume than tea and coffee and, although tea dominates, cultural choices are usually polarised: coffee in America and Europe, tea in England and Asia. It is likely that caffeine, the world's most popular psychoactive drug, is the core of their day-to-day appeal, but their anti-inflammatory polyphenols are the stimulus that matters most.

7   Li, X., Yu, C., Guo, Y., et al. (2017). Tea consumption and risk of ischaemic heart disease. *Heart*, 103(10), 783-789
8   Peters, U., Poole, C., & Arab, L. (2001). Does tea affect cardiovascular disease? A meta-analysis. *American Journal of Epidemiology*, 154(6), 495-503.
9   Arab, L., Liu, W., & Elashoff, D. (2009). Green and black tea consumption and risk of stroke: a meta-analysis. *Stroke*, 40(5), 1786-92.
10 Feng, L., Li, J., Ng, T., Lee, T., Kua, E., & Zeng, Y. (2013). Tea drinking and cognitive function in oldest-old Chinese. *The Journal of Nutrition, Health & Aging*, 16(9), 754-758.
11 Ruan, R., Feng, L., Li, J., Ng, T., & Zeng, Y. (2013). Tea Consumption and Mortality in the Oldest-Old Chinese. *Journal of American Geriatrics Society*, 61(11), 1937-1942.

References

Arab, L., Liu, W., & Elashoff, D. (2009). Green and black tea consumption and risk of stroke: a meta-analysis. *Stroke*, 40(5), 1786-92.

Bae, J-H., Park, J-H., Im, S-S., & Song, D-K. (2014). Coffee and health. *Integrative Medicine Research*, 3(4), 189-191.

Bai, W., Wang, C., & Ren, C. (2014). Intakes of total and individual flavonoids by US adults. *International Journal of Food Sciences & Nutrition*, 65(1), 9-20.

Bøhn, S., Blomhoff, R., & Paur, I. (2014). Coffee and cancer risk, epidemiological evidence, and molecular mechanisms. *Molecular Nutrition & Food Research*, 58(5), 915-930.

Chrysant, S. (2015). Coffee Consumption and Cardiovascular Health. *The American Journal of Cardiology*, 116(5), 818-821.

Das, M., Sur, P., Gomes, A., Vedasiromoni, J., & Ganguly, D. (2002). Inhibition of tumour growth and inflammation by consumption of tea. *Phytotherapy Research*, 16(S1), 40-44.

Ding, M., Satija, A., Bhupathiraju, S.N., et al. (2015). Association of Coffee Consumption with Total and Cause-Specific Mortality in Three Large Prospective Cohorts. *Circulation*, 132(24), 2305-2315.

Dufresne, C., & Farnworth, E. (2000). Tea, Kombucha, and health: a review. *Food Research International*, 33(6), 409-421.

Feng, L., Li, J., Ng, T., Lee, T., Kua, E., & Zeng, Y. (2013). Tea drinking and cognitive function in oldest-old Chinese. *The Journal of Nutrition, Health & Aging*, 16(9), 754-758.

Gaascht, F., Dicato, M., & Diederich, M. (2015). Coffee provides a natural multitarget pharmacopeia against the hallmarks of cancer. *Genes & Nutrition*, 10(6), 1-17.

Grigg, D. (2002). The worlds of tea and coffee: Patterns of consumption. *GeoJournal*, 57(4), 283-294.

Hodgson, J., & Croft, K. (2010). Tea flavonoids and cardiovascular health. *Molecular Aspects of Medicine*, 31(6), 495-502.

Jiang, W., Wu, Y., & Jiang, X. (2013). Coffee and caffeine intake and breast cancer risk: An updated dose–response meta-analysis of 37 published studies. *Gynecologic Oncology*, 129(3), 620-629.

Larsson, S., Virtamo, J., & Wolk, A. (2013). Black tea consumption and risk of stroke in women and men. *Annals of Epidemiology*, 23(3), 157-160.

Lee, M., McGeer, E., & McGeer, P. (2016). Quercetin, not caffeine, is a major neuroprotective component in coffee. *Neurobiology of Aging*, 46, 113-123.

Li, X., Yu, C., Guo, Y., et al. (2017). Tea consumption and risk of ischaemic heart disease. *Heart*, 103(10), 783-789.

Liang, N., & Kitts, D.D. (2016). Role of Chlorogenic Acids in Controlling Oxidative and Inflammatory Stress Conditions. *Nutrients*, 8(1), 16.

Liu, S., Zheng, H., Sun, R., Jiang, H., Chen, J., Yu, J., Zhang, Q., Chen, Q., Zhu, L., Hu, M., Lu, L., & Liu, Z. (2017). Disposition of Flavonoids for Personal Intake. *Current Pharmacology Reports*, 3(4), 196-212.

Ludwig, I., Clifford, M., Lean, M., Ashihara, H., & Crozier, A. (2014). Coffee: biochemistry and potential impact on health. *Food & Function*, 5(8), 1695-1717.

Miller, P., Zhao, D., Frazier-Wood, A., Michos, E., Averill, M., Sandfort, V., Burke, G., Polak, J., Lima, J., Post, W., Blumenthal, R., Guallar, E., & Martin, S. (2017). Associations of Coffee, Tea, and Caffeine Intake with Coronary Artery Calcification and Cardiovascular Events. *The American Journal of Medicine*, 130(2), 188-197.e5.

Mo, H., Zhu, Y., & Chen, Z. (2008). Microbial fermented tea – a potential source of natural food preservatives. *Trends in Food Science & Technology*, 19(3), 124-130.

Park, S., Freedman, N.D., Haiman, C.A., Le Marchand, L., Wilkens, L.R., & Setiawan, V.W. (2017). Association of Coffee Consumption With Total and Cause-Specific Mortality Among Nonwhite Populations. *Annals of Internal Medicine*.

Peters, U., Poole, C., & Arab, L. (2001). Does tea affect cardiovascular disease? A meta-analysis. *American Journal of Epidemiology*, 154(6), 495-503.

Peterson, J., Dwyer, J., Bhagwat, S., Haytowitz, D., Holden, J., Eldridge, A., Beecher, G., & Aladesanmi, J. (2005). Major flavonoids in dry tea. *Journal of Food Composition and Analysis*, 18(6), 487-501.

Pourshahidi, L., Navarini, L., Petracco, M., & Strain, J. (2016). A Comprehensive Overview of the Risks and Benefits of Coffee Consumption. *Comprehensive Reviews in Food Science and Food Safety*, 15(4), 671-684.

Ruan, R., Feng, L., Li, J., Ng, T., & Zeng, Y. (2013). Tea Consumption and Mortality in the Oldest-Old Chinese. *Journal of American Geriatrics Society*, 61(11), 1937-1942.

Ruxton, H.C. (2009). The health effects of black tea and flavonoids. *Nutrition & Food Science*, 39(3), 283-294.

Saab, S., Mallam, D., & Cox, G. Impact of coffee on liver diseases: a systematic review. *Liver International*, 34(4) 1478-3231.

Svilaas, A., Sakhi, A., Andersen, L., Svilaas, T., Ström, E., Jacobs, D., Ose, L., & Blomhoff, R. (2004). Intakes of Antioxidants in Coffee, Wine, and Vegetables Are Correlated with Plasma Carotenoids in Humans. *The Journal of Nutrition*, 134(3), 562

Taguchi, C., Fukushima, Y., Kishimoto, Y., et al. (2015). Estimated Dietary Polyphenol Intake and Major Food and Beverage Sources among Elderly Japanese. *Nutrients*, 7(12), 10269-10281.

Temple, J.L., Bernard, C., Lipshultz, S.E., Czachor, J.D., Westphal, J.A., & Mestre, M.A. (2017). The Safety of Ingested Caffeine: A Comprehensive Review. *Frontiers in Psychiatry*, 8, 80.

Torres, D. (2013). Is It Time to Write a Prescription for Coffee? Coffee and Liver Disease. *Gastroenterology*, 144(4), 670-672.

Wierzejska, R. (2017). Can coffee consumption lower the risk of Alzheimer's disease and Parkinson's disease? A literature review. *Archives of Medical Science : AMS*, 13(3), 507-514.

Yashin, A., Yashin, Y., Wang, J.Y., & Nemzer, B. (2013). Antioxidant and Antiradical Activity of Coffee. *Antioxidants*, 2(4), 230-245.

Zamora-Ros, R., Rothwell, J.A., Scalbert, A., et al. (2013). Dietary intakes and food sources of phenolic acids in the European Prospective Investigation into Cancer and Nutrition (EPIC) study. *British Journal of Nutrition*, 110(8), 1500-11.

27

CEREAL KILLERS
The right and wrong way to eat grain

There is one simple thing to be said about grain food: it is good for you in its original packaging, and bad for you when deconstructed. In other words, whole grains are healthy, and white flour is not. The difference is vital, as grain is humanity's largest source of calories, and has been ever since prehistoric nomads got fed up with foraging and planted their own seeding grass. The human race founded civilisation on grain, and without it there would be no modern world. Yet the modern world has wrought havoc on our daily bread, sending the best part for cattle food, or industrial alcohol, and feeding humans the residue.

The first evidence for whole grains came from the *British Medical Journal*, which reported that, in a group of three hundred London men, the whole-grain eaters had healthier hearts.[1] That was in 1977, and numerous studies have since confirmed it: people who eat all their grains have fewer inflammatory conditions like heart disease, diabetes or cancer. The benefit eludes people who eat only the starchy bit, which means the divisions within a wheat berry, of which there are three, are not created equal.

---

1   Morris, J. N., Marr, J. W., & Clayton, D. G. (1977). Diet and heart: a postscript. *British Medical Journal*, 2(6098), 1307-14.

The outer layer of a kernel of grain is fibrous. It holds everything together and protects it like a shell. This is bran. Within is the germ, the embryo, which grows into a new plant with warmth and water, and between the two is the endosperm. The endosperm is a padding of starch and it is endosperm that gives us white flour. It is a culinary tragedy of the first order that white flour is so palatable, as the endosperm is not where the true nutrition lies. Most bread and pasta are white flour and are not much better for your health than eating sugar lumps.

Like fruit and vegetables, grain is rich in antioxidants such as folates, carotenoids, and phenolic acids, all of which sweep up free radicals, and prod genes to make internal antioxidant enzymes. Some of the highest polyphenol counts come from unusual grain like buckwheat and quinoa[2] which outrank wheat and rice by a large margin. Also, several particularly potent antioxidants, like ferulic acid, are grain monopolies. In other words, grain is the only effective way of getting them. Authorities see the polyphenols from fruit and grain as synergistic, meaning it is the range rather than total number that packs the punch. An optimal polyphenol load does not rest entirely on fruit and vegetables, which should give pause to the anti-carbohydrate lobby. Whole grains also have impressive levels of vitamin E – a potent, free-radical scavenger – various B vitamins, and trace metals like zinc and magnesium which are essential constituents of antioxidant enzymes.

By far the highest fraction of phytochemicals resides in the germ and bran, which is why good health means the whole kernel. That doesn't necessarily mean eating grains in their wholly natural state. Grains are crushed, cracked or boiled before they are eaten, as they would be difficult to chew if they were not, and *whole grain* means keeping

---

2   Strictly speaking buckwheat and quinoa are seeds but not cereals as they come from broadleaf plants and not grasses. The distinction is not significant for culinary purposes.

the different parts together, even if they are processed in some way. Porridge, when made with whole rolled oat groats, is a whole-grain food, as is bread made from whole-grain flour; also coloured rice (not the white stuff), or any other boiled seed like quinoa. Food vendors like to play on the whole grain concept and have an innovative range of adjectives to mislead the unwary. 'Multi-grain' and 'stone ground' labels make you think of seed heads bobbing in the wind, even if the bread they are stuck on is starchy pap rendered brown with coffee (yes, really). The only term that means whole grain is whole grain, and innocent fun can be had spotting labels that dance on a pin head to avoid it.

However, not all technology is detrimental. Even traditionally milled grain has its drawbacks since bran is tough and fibrous and binds its phytochemicals so they do not absorb well from the gut. Incidentally, this is a happy state of affairs for the gut which gets to hold onto the phytochemicals and pass them along. That may well be why whole grains protect against bowel cancer. In the interests of making the phytochemicals available to a wider audience, food scientists have given thought to ways of making the bran more cooperative. Ultrafine grinding seems to work, as smaller particles are easier for bowel bacteria to break down, and commercial enzymes can be added to assist. Sprouting grain before milling it plays on the seed's biology as sprouting unbinds nutrients for the shoot to consume. Sprouting is also within reach of the home kitchen and renders grain edible without cooking.

Alternatively, some health-motivated millers address the issue by adding extra bran; others, even more innovatively, selectively fortify flour with the best bits to render their product nutritionally superior to its original ingredients. The richest seam in the bran shell is the innermost aleurone layer, and modern microcontrolled abrasion techniques can peel it away and concentrate it. The ultimate marriage of tradition and science is separating microparticles of bran with an electric field, as the particles with the most ferulic acid have the highest positive charge and can be dragged out. Much of this remains the preserve of laboratories, not bakeries, particularly as bran fortification undermines taste and texture, and requires further chemical tweaks to retain palatability. But the techniques are marching forward on multiple fronts so that flour, or at least some of its iterations, can become healthier, which means it can become more anti-inflammatory.

So choose your daily bread carefully. It can be pro- or anti-inflammatory, and it can be neutered or enriched in that direction by the hands it has passed through, and their take on modern milling. A critical and well-informed eye is called for. Antagonising inflammation also means eating some of the less common cereals and reserving a regular dietary niche for sprouted ones. But wherever or whatever, whole is the goal.

References

Anson, N., Hemery, Y., Bast, A., & Haenen, G. (2012). Optimizing the bioactive potential of wheat bran by processing. *Food & Function,* 3(4), 362-375.

Bhupathiraju, S., & Tucker, K. (2011). Coronary heart disease prevention: Nutrients, foods, and dietary patterns. *Clinica Chimica Acta,* 412(17), 1493-1514.

Björck, I., Östman, E., Kristensen, M., Mateo Anson, N., Price, R., Haenen, G., Havenaar, R., Bach Knudsen, K., Frid, A., Mykkänen, H., Welch, R., & Riccardi, G. (2012). Cereal grains for nutrition and health benefits: Overview of results from in vitro , animal and human studies in the HEALTHGRAIN project. *Trends in Food Science & Technology,* 25(2), 87-100.

Brewer, L., Kubola, J., Siriamornpun, S., Herald, T., & Shi, Y. (2014). Wheat bran particle size influence on phytochemical extractability and antioxidant properties. *Food Chemistry,* 152, 483-490.

Fardet, A., Rock, E., & Rémésy, C. (2008). Is the in vitro antioxidant potential of whole-grain cereals and cereal products well reflected in vivo? *Journal of Cereal Science,* 48(2), 258-276.

Gage, F. (2006). Wheat into Flour: A Story of Milling. Gastronomica: *The Journal of Food and Culture,* 6(1).

Gorinstein, S., Vargas, O., Jaramillo, N., Salas, I., Ayala, A., Arancibia-Avila, P., Toledo, F., Katrich, E., & Trakhtenberg, S. (2007). The total polyphenols and the antioxidant potentials of some selected cereals and pseudocereals. *European Food Research and Technology,* 225(3), 321-328.

Grigor, J., Brennan, C., Hutchings, S., & Rowlands, D. (2016). The sensory acceptance of fibre-enriched cereal foods: a meta-analysis. *International Journal of Food Science & Technology,* 51(1), 3-13.

Hemery, Y., Rouau, X., Lullien-Pellerin, V., Barron, C., & Abecassis, J. (2007). Dry processes to develop wheat fractions and products with enhanced nutritiona l quality. *Journal of Cereal Science,* 46(3), 327-347.

Lee, Y., Han, S., Song, B., & Yeum, K. (2015). Bioactives in Commonly Consumed Cereal Grains: Implications for Oxidative Stress and Inflammation. *Journal of Medicinal Food.*

Liu, R. (2007). Whole grain phytochemicals and health. *Journal of Cereal Science,* 46(3), 207-219.

Morris, J. N., Marr, J. W., & Clayton, D. G. (1977). Diet and heart: a postscript. *British Medical Journal,* 2(6098), 1307-14.

Palmarola-Adrados, B., Chotěborská, P., Galbe, M., & Zacchi, G. (2005). Ethanol production from non-starch carbohydrates of wheat bran. *Bioresource Technology,* 96(7), 843-850.

28

RUN FOR YOUR LIFE

The universal imperative to move

Through every epoch of human development, survival has meant exertion. Whether it was hunting the woolly mammoth, or ploughing the Nile valley, or labouring in the mines and factories of the industrial revolution, humans have always been creatures of activity, and we have been formed to last longer when we live that way. Unfortunately, at least for our health, we now have engines, and the manifold marvels of electricity. Today a workout is reserved for the sports field, and the average citizen thinks a walk around the block is a major concession to wellness. We are the first people in history who can choose not to exercise, and our well-being is in crisis because of it.

The issue was first officially spotted in 1953, when the English medical journal The Lancet reported that London bus conductors had less heart disease than the drivers.[1] It also reported the same finding for postmen compared to telephone operators. The observation has been made many times and in many different ways since. Our bodies last longer when we move them, but they become inflamed with cancer, diabetes and heart disease when we do not.

---

1   Morris, J.N., Heady, J.A., Raffle, P.A., Roberts, C.G., & Parks, J.W. (1953). Coronary heart-disease and physical activity of work. *Lancet*, 65(6795), 1053-1057.

Despite this, most adults do not get enough exercise to reap its benefits. Inactivity compares with smoking and processed food as a simple, common and avoidable cause of premature illness and death, but the message is not being heeded.

Exertion as minimal as gardening and using the stairs is effective. Walking an extra 15 minutes a day – about a mile – wards off heart attacks and adds years to life. Even people who start exercising when they are elderly can fend off illness and push out their lifespan. Exercise trumps body weight, in that obese people who exercise do better than normal weight people who sit around. Perhaps the greatest evidence of its physiological super status is that exercise treats some cases of diseases, like diabetes, as well as drugs do.

Exercise improves various things like weight and blood pressure, but central among them is inflammation. Blood-borne markers of inflammation are lower in people who exercise regularly, and there are various reasons why. Exercise releases white cells into the blood, but suppresses their function. There are more of them, but they have fewer teeth.

More obviously, exercise burns fat, which is inflammatory (see The fire in the fat). In particular, exercise breaks up fat around organs like the liver, which is the most dangerous type, and will eat away at such fat even when it is not changing body weight. Exercise also damps down the cytokines that fat deposits secrete, and stops white blood cells invading them, which is an important part of the inflammatory process.

Cytokines also have a lot to do with muscles. Everyone has recently been surprised to discover that muscles do more than just power joints: they modify surrounding inflammation with their own in-house brand of cytokines. Such cytokines are called myokines, and myokines seem to deliver a lot of exercise's benefits. Key myokines can increase 100-fold in the blood with sustained exercise, and myokines modify inflammation at distant sites.

Exercise also causes stress. It makes the body work and the heart pump faster. Stress releases hormones like adrenaline and cortisol, which are helpful vis-à-vis inflammation because they contain it. Healthy inflammation that repels infections and repairs injuries flares up where the problem is, but needs to be restrained elsewhere, so the system releases hormones to ring-fence it. When the nervous system records stress, these hormones course through the bloodstream and hose down everything beyond the combat zone. But hormone responses are blunt, not fine-tuned. They do not know if the stress signals are from an inflammatory event or not. That means controlled non-toxic stress, such as a good run, floods the system with natural anti-inflammatories.

This also helps explain why exercise can sometimes be overdone. Inflammation is a good thing when it is fighting a virus or healing a cut, but ring-fencing hormones do not discriminate. Because of them, people who overdo exercise suffer more infections, and their wounds heal more slowly. However, the ceiling is high, and the foregoing is not a note of caution. Most people would be better off doing more than they usually do, particularly walking.

Exercise expends energy. Pumping muscles chew through much more energy than resting ones, which is one of the reasons people prod themselves into it so they can lose weight. As per The inflammage, burning food throws off unstable molecules called free radicals, so there are more after exercise. Free radicals are inflammatory stimulants and serious killers of normal cell structures, which implies more should be harmful. But there is a paradox in play. Cells run complex antioxidant systems to deal with free radicals, and robust antioxidant defences are key anti-inflammatory, long-life promoting consequences of healthy lifestyle choices. When more free radicals come down the pipeline, in manageable bursts, they give the antioxidant systems a boost. The net effect is a benefit: more free radicals, but better ways of dealing with them. People who sit around all day have more free radicals in their organs than people who exercise, despite making fewer of them—the difference is the tuning of their removal machinery.

Exercise also makes more mitochondria, the cell furnaces that burn food. Mitochondria get slow and tatty as you get older, and a lot of research ties tatty mitochondria with the ravages of age, and its big diseases. Exercise prods the activity of genes that make a protein called PGC1α – even a single bout of exercise releases a spike of it – which regulates antioxidant defences in various ways. In particular, it tells the mitochondria to copy themselves, and turn out shiny new ones.

One way of looking at it is that exercise is not healthy: it stretches, strains and exhausts the body and pumps out poisons. It is the recovery that is healthy. Exercise causes adaptation. When the insults are regular, the response becomes disciplined. It is not just muscles that bulk up. So do the anti-inflammatory responses.

References

Booth, F.W., Roberts, C.K., & Laye, M.J. (2012). Lack of exercise is a major cause of chronic diseases. *Comprehensive Physiology,* 2(2), 1143-1211.

Buresh, R., & Berg, K. (2015). A tutorial on oxidative stress and redox signaling with application to exercise and sedentariness. *Sports Medicine - Open,* 1(1), 1-9.

Chen, Y., Fredericson, M., Matheson, G., & Phillips, E. (2013). Exercise is Medicine. *Current Physical Medicine and Rehabilitation Reports,* 1(1), 48-56.

Chung, H.Y., Cesari, M., Anton, S., et al. (2009). Molecular Inflammation: Underpinnings of Aging and Age-related Diseases. *Ageing Research Reviews,* 8(1), 18-30.

Coppotelli, G., & Ross, J.M. (2016). Mitochondria in Ageing and Diseases: The Super Trouper of the Cell *International Journal of Molecular Sciences,* 17(5), 711.

Das, U. (2004). Anti-inflammatory nature of exercise. *Nutrition,* 20(3), 323-326.

Eijsvogels, T., Molossi, S., Lee, D., Emery, M., & Thompson, P. (2016). Exercise at the Extremes. *Journal of the American College of Cardiology*, 67(3), 316-329.

Handschin, C., & Spiegelman, B. (2008). The role of exercise and PGC1α in inflammation and chronic disease. *Nature*, 454(7203), 463-469.

Koelwyn, G.J., Wennerberg, E., Demaria, S., & Jones, L.W. (2015). Exercise in Regulation of Inflammation-Immune Axis Function in Cancer Initiation and Progression. *Oncology (Williston Park, NY)*, 29(12), 214800.

Lewis, S., & Hennekens, C. (2016). Regular Physical Activity: Forgotten Benefits. *The American Journal of Medicine*, 129(2), 137-138.

Morris, J.N., Heady, J.A., Raffle, P.A., Roberts, C.G., & Parks, J.W. (1953). Coronary heart-disease and physical activity of work. *Lancet*, 65(6795), 1053-1057.

Newton, R., & Galvão, D. (2008). Exercise in Prevention and Management of Cancer. *Current Treatment Options in Oncology*, 9(2), 135-146.

Nimmo, M. A., Leggate, M., Viana, J.L. & King, J.A. (2013). The effect of physical activity on mediators of inflammation. *Diabetes Obesity & Metabolism*, 15(3), 51-60.

Petersen, A., & Pedersen, B. (2005). The anti-inflammatory effect of exercise. *Journal of Applied Physiology*, 98(4), 1154.

Phillips, S.A., Mahmoud, A.M., Brown, M.D., & Haus, J.M. (2015). Exercise Interventions and Peripheral Arterial Function: Implications for Cardio-Metabolic Disease. *Progress in Cardiovascular Diseases*, 57(5), 521-534.

Powers, S., Radak, Z., & Ji, L. (2016). Exercise-induced oxidative stress: past, present and future. *The Journal of Physiology*, 594(18), 5081-5092.

Radak, Z., Chung, H., Koltai, E., Taylor, A., & Goto, S. (2008). Exercise, oxidative stress and hormesis. *Ageing Research Reviews*, 7(1), 34-42.

Schnyder, S., & Handschin, C. (2015). Skeletal muscle as an endocrine organ: PGC-1α, myokines and exercise. *Bone*, 80, 115-125.

Simon, H. (2015). Exercise and Health: Dose and Response, Considering Both Ends of the Curve. *The American Journal of Medicine*, 128(11), 1171-1177.

Smith, L. (2012). Overtraining, Excessive Exercise, and Altered Immunity. *Sports Medicine*, 33(5), 347-364.

Viña, J., Gomez-Cabrera, M., Borras, C., Froio, T., Sanchis-Gomar, F., Martinez-Bello, V., & Pallardo, F. (2009). Mitochondrial biogenesis in exercise and in ageing. *Advanced Drug Delivery Reviews*, 61(14), 1369-1374.

Vollaard, N., Shearman, J., & Cooper, C. (2012). Exercise-Induced Oxidative Stress. *Sports Medicine*, 35(12), 1045-1062.

Wen, C., Wai, J., Tsai, M., & Chen, C. (2014). Minimal Amount of Exercise to Prolong Life. *Journal of the American College of Cardiology*, 64(5), 482-484.

29

SPICE OF LIFE

Soothing effects of pepper and herbs

Turmeric, as we have seen, is a standout, natural anti-inflammatory and one of the most widely used spices in the world. However, despite its remarkable properties, it is not unique. There are many other preserving and flavouring plants that show anti-inflammatory promise, particularly when traditional cuisines in which they figure, like the ones in Asia and the Mediterranean, are picked apart. Spices are rich sources of polyphenol anti-inflammatories, as are herbs, and both of them compare with the best of fruit and vegetables. The question is whether their polyphenols make a difference in the tiny quantities that people eat. The answer, perhaps surprisingly, is that they probably do.

Chronic diseases like cancer are less common in Asia than the modern West, and diet is likely to be part of the reason. One of the distinctive differences between Asian and Western eating is spices. Chilli peppers are a good start. The eye-watering burn comes from a molecule called capsaicin which, despite what it does to the lining of your mouth, actually soothes inflammation. Chilli pepper is a major force in Chinese food and, since 2004, a large study in China has followed the health of half a million subjects. According to *The BMJ*,[1]

---

1   The British Medical Journal changed its name to just 'The BMJ' in 1988.

it found that 'The habitual consumption of spicy foods was inversely associated with total and certain cause specific mortality (cancer, ischaemic heart disease and respiratory disease).'[2]

In other words, spicy-food eaters did not die as often during the study period and, when they did, it was less likely to be from major inflammatory conditions like cancer and heart disease.

Some research suggests stomach cancer is an exception and that spicy diets increase the risk, possibly because direct irritation of the stomach lining, a known cause of cancer, overwhelms the anti-inflammatory effect. The result of this Chinese study shows this is less significant than the number of cancers prevented.

The effect of chilli in population studies is mirrored in laboratory findings. In one study, irritants were injected into the lung and abdominal linings of anaesthetised rats, some of whom were dosed beforehand with juice from red peppers.[3] When they were euthanised, and their lining membranes examined under a microscope, membranes from the treated rats had fewer inflammatory white blood cells and less permeable blood vessels (recall inflammation runs off leaky blood vessels, see Inflammation, nuts and bolts). They also had fewer inflammatory cytokines. Further observations implied capsaicin was responsible. Various laboratory models show capsaicin is potentially effective for suppressing cancers of bowel, lung and prostate.

As discussed in Keeping the lines open, the reaction of blood-borne particles of cholesterol with oxygen is a key step that makes cholesterol irritate the immune system, and provoke the inflammation that underpins heart disease. There is evidence the reaction can be

---

2 Lv, J., Qi, L., Yu, C., et al. (2015). Consumption of spicy foods and total and cause specific mortality: population based cohort study. *The BMJ*, 351, h3942.
3 Spiller, F., Alves, M., Vieira, S., Carvalho, T., Leite, C., Lunardelli, A., Poloni, J., Cunha, F., & Oliveira, J. (2008). Anti-inflammatory effects of red pepper (Capsicum baccatum) on carrageenan- and antigen-induced inflammation. *Journal of Pharmacy and Pharmacology: An International Journal of Pharmaceutical Science*, 60(4).

stopped by capsaicin, as well as curcumin from turmeric, quercetin from garlic, eugenol from cloves and piperine, the active ingredient in black pepper.

Doctors regularly treat pain with capsaicin. Capsaicin cream is particularly good for nerve pain and its effects have a lot to do with a structure called the TRPV1 receptor. The TRPV1 receptor is a gatekeeper found in many organs, particularly the brain and nerves, through which toxins like chemicals and heat stir up pain and inflammation.

Cinnamon is another major player. The name means 'sweet wood' and the familiar quills are tree bark, which curls up when it dries. Among various active ingredients, inhibiting inflammation seems to rest mainly with cinnamaldehyde, which seems particularly effective for inflammation in the brain. Neuroinflammation, as it is called, lies behind some big diseases like Parkinson's and Alzheimer's. Cinnamaldehyde is a powerful inhibitor of inflammation associated with microglia, which are the brain's specialist immune cells. It also shows promise in treating laboratory animals affected by arthritis.

Cinnamon, like cloves, also yields the polyphenol eugenol. Eugenol inhibits multiple inflammatory signals, and early data suggests it can modify asthma, atherosclerosis and cancer. In laboratory conditions, it can even assist conventional cancer drugs.

Herbs, which are leaves – while spices are everything else like bark and seeds – are much the same. Some experts think there may be more to the Mediterranean diet than tomatoes and sardines, and that part of its long-life benefit comes from the herbs, like rosemary and oregano, that often figure. One study compared the diets of people who were admitted to a major hospital in Rome with lung cancer, with well people of the same age.[4] It found that in addition to the expected items

---

4   Fortes, C., Forastiere, F., Farchi, S., Mallone, S., Trequattrinni, T., Anatra, F., Schmid, G., & Perucci, C.A. (2003). The protective effect of the Mediterranean diet on lung cancer. *Nutrition And Cancer*, 46(1), 30-7.

of good eating, like carrots and olive oil, the well people also ate more herbs, particularly sage.

One of the key herbal polyphenols is rosemarinic acid. Rosemarinic acid was first found in rosemary, obviously, and has since been found in numerous other common herbs like oregano, parsley and mint. Rosemarinic acid interferes with NF-κB and various genes that code for specialised inflammatory proteins (see Epigenetics, and food as information). When rosemarinic acid is administered to mice with inflamed lungs (an artificial model of asthma), inflammatory cells, mucous and thickened membranes – all part of asthma – are alleviated.[5]

Carnosic acid, another anti-inflammatory from rosemary, affects cytokine levels and multiple other inflammatory mechanisms in fat cells, particularly those from laboratory rats that are obese. A derivative called carnosol, also found in sage, has been shown in laboratory settings to inhibit multiple models of cancer, including prostate, breast and skin.

As per The inflammage, ageing tends to mean too many free radicals and too few enzymes to remove them. One of the most important of those enzymes, superoxide dismutase, is enhanced by the polyphenols in rosemary, sage and thyme, and the effect persists even after they have been cooked. Parsley, both fresh and cooked, also increased blood levels of various antioxidant enzymes in a laboratory setting.

Basil, fenugreek, coriander and all the others can tell similar stories. Kitchens from Calcutta to Crete have spent millennia enriching their eating with the standout flavours of the plant world, and modern evidence implies a robust anti-inflammatory lifestyle lies in emulating them.

---

5 Rocha, J., Eduardo-Figueira, M., Barateiro, A., Fernandes, A., Brites, D., Bronze, R., Duarte, C., Serra, A., Pinto, R., Freitas, M., Fernandes, E., Silva-Lima, B., Mota-Filipe, H., & Sepodes, B. (2015). Anti-inflammatory Effect of Rosmarinic Acid and an Extract of Rosmarinus officinalis in Rat Models of Local and Systemic Inflammation. *Basic and Clinical Pharmacology & Toxicology*, 116(5), 398-413.

References

Akhilender Naidu, K., & Thippeswamy, N. (2004). Inhibition of human low density lipoprotein oxidation by active principles from spices. *Molecular and Cellular Biochemistry,* 229(2), 19-23.

Chen, Y.-H., Zou, X.-N., Zheng, T.-Z., et al. (2017). High Spicy Food Intake and Risk of Cancer: A Meta-analysis of Case–control Studies. *Chinese Medical Journal,* 130(18), 2241-2250.

Chohan, M., Naughton, D., & Opara, E. (2014). Determination of superoxide dismutase mimetic activity in common culinary herbs. *SpringerPlus,* 3(1), 1-4.

Dragland, S., Senoo, H., Wake, K., Holte, K., & Blomhoff, R. (2003). Several culinary and medicinal herbs are important sources of dietary antioxidants. *Journal of Nutrition,* 133(5), 1286-90.

Fortes, C., Forastiere, F., Farchi, S., Mallone, S., Trequattrinni, T., Anatra, F., Schmid, G., & Perucci, C.A. (2003). The protective effect of the Mediterranean diet on lung cancer. *Nutrition and Cancer,* 46(1), 30-7.

Gawlik-Dziki, U. (2012). Dietary spices as a natural effectors of lipoxygenase, xanthine oxidase, peroxidase and antioxidant agents. *LWT - Food Science and Technology,* 47(1), 138-146.

Hassani, F., Shirani, K., & Hosseinzadeh, H. (2016). Rosemary (Rosmarinus officinalis) as a potential therapeutic plant in metabolic syndrome: a review. *Naunyn-Schmiedeberg's Archives of Pharmacology,* 389(9), 931-949.

Ho, S., Chang, K., & Chang, P. (2013). Inhibition of neuroinflammation by cinnamon and its main components. *Food Chemistry,* 138(4), 2275-2282.

Hostetler, G., Ralston, R., & Schwartz, S. (2017). Flavones: Food Sources, Bioavailability, Metabolism, and Bioactivity. *Advances in Nutrition,* 8(3), 423-435.

Johnson, J. (2011). Carnosol: A promising anti-cancer and anti-inflammatory agent. *Cancer Letters,* 305(1), 1-7.

Kannappan, R., Gupta, S.C., Kim, J.H., Reuter, S., & Aggarwal, B.B. (2011). Neuroprotection by Spice-Derived Nutraceuticals: You Are What You Eat! *Molecular Neurobiology,* 44(2), 142-159.

Kaul, P., Bhattacharya, A., Rajeswara Rao, B., Syamasundar, K., & Ramesh, S. (2003). Volatile constituents of essential oils isolated from different parts of cinnamon (Cinnamomum zeylanicum Blume). *Journal of the Science of Food and Agriculture,* 83(1), 53-55.

Kunnumakkara, A.B., Sailo, B.L., Banik, K., et al. (2018). Chronic diseases, inflammation, and spices: how are they linked? *Journal of Translational Medicine,* 16, 14.

Lv, J., Qi, L., Yu, C., et al. (2015). Consumption of spicy foods and total and cause specific mortality: population based cohort study. *The BMJ,* 351, h3942.

Opara, E.I., & Chohan, M. (2014). Culinary herbs and spices: their bioactive properties, the contribution of polyphenols and the challenges in deducing their true health benefits. *International Journal of Molecular Science,* 15(10), 19183-202.

Rafehi, H., Ververis, K., & Karagiannis, T. (2012). Controversies surrounding the clinical potential of cinnamon for the management of diabetes. *Diabetes Obesity & Metabolism,* 14(6).

Rocha, J., Eduardo-Figueira, M., Barateiro, A., Fernandes, A., Brites, D., Bronze, R., Duarte, C., Serra, A., Pinto, R., Freitas, M., Fernandes, E., Silva-Lima, B., Mota-Filipe, H., & Sepodes, B. (2015). Anti-inflammatory Effect of Rosmarinic Acid and an Extract of Rosmarinus officinalis in Rat Models of Local and Systemic Inflammation. *Basic and Clinical Pharmacology & Toxicology,* 116(5), 398-413.

Spiller, F., Alves, M., Vieira, S., Carvalho, T., Leite, C., Lunardelli, A., Poloni, J., Cunha, F., & Oliveira, J. (2008). Anti-inflammatory effects of red pepper (Capsicum baccatum) on carrageenan- and antigen-induced inflammation. *Journal of Pharmacy and Pharmacology: An International Journal of Pharmaceutical Science,* 60(4).

Sun, F., Xiong, S., & Zhu, Z. (2016). Dietary Capsaicin Protects Cardiometabolic Organs from Dysfunction. *Nutrients,* 8(5), 174.

Sung, B., Prasad, S., Yadav, V.R., & Aggarwal, B.B. (2012). Cancer Cell Signaling Pathways Targeted by Spice-Derived Nutraceuticals. *Nutrition and Cancer,* 64(2), 173-197.

Veronesi, B., & Oortgiesen, M. (2006). The TRPV1 Receptor: Target of Toxicants and Therapeutics. *Toxicological Sciences,* 89(1), 1-3.

Yashin, A., Yashin, Y., Xia, X., & Nemzer, B. (2017). Antioxidant Activity of Spices and Their Impact on Human Health: A Review. *Antioxidants (Basel),* 6(3), 70.

30

ASIA'S ANCIENT PROTEIN
The versatile soy bean

Soy beans have been a staple in Asia since Chinese farmers domesticated them, which archaeologists say happened at least three millennia ago. Soy took a while to catch on when it arrived in the West in the eighteenth century, but it exploded in importance in the twentieth, because of its unique adaptability. Soy traditionally comes as milk and miso, tempeh and tofu, and Asian cuisine's signature fermented sauce. The same versatility proved ideal for industrial food, and now it turns up in every aisle of the supermarket: bread and breakfast cereals, pasta and yoghurt, processed meat and its animal-free substitutes – like vegetarian sausages and hamburgers – tinned tuna and a thousand items more.

Soy was one of the first foods to be called 'functional', probably because that movement began in Japan. Unusual among plants, it is a 'complete' protein, like meat, which means it contains all nine amino acids your body can't manufacture. It is also high in fibre. Soy did not get off to a good start when food scientists first probed it. Soy is the human diet's richest source of molecules called isoflavones which, it was discovered in the 1940s, cause infertility in sheep that ate red clover. Isoflavones are a type of polyphenol called phytoestrogens – which refers to oestrogens from plants – because they mimic the hormone oestrogen. Certain cancers, like breast, can be hormone-sensitive, so eating hormones, even plant versions, doesn't sound like a good idea. For several decades there was debate, fuelled by some animal studies which showed harm, about whether isoflavones were good or bad. Modern insights show laboratory animals, even primates, metabolise soy isoflavones very differently from humans. The consensus is that human population studies are more useful than animal experiments in this area, which is fortunate as human studies consistently show soy is safe and useful, at least in whole food or its traditionally processed form.[1] The remnants of this debate still survive in corners of the Internet, although major authorities like the European Food Safety Authority and the American Cancer Society consistently say soy isoflavones are safe.

In fact, population studies have found far less cancer of the breast, prostate and uterus in countries where people eat a lot of soy.[2] At the risk of oversimplifying a complex subject, the point seems to be that isoflavones block oestrogen receptors more than they stimulate them, like a key that enters a lock but doesn't turn it. Breast cancer drugs do much the same.

Isoflavones, like all phytochemicals, have multiple targets not just hormonal ones. A lot of evidence shows soy lowers cholesterol and blood pressure, albeit modestly, but enough to improve the incidence of heart disease when a whole population eat it. Soy-consuming parts of the planet have less cardiovascular disease, and this is at least part of the reason why.

Soy may help with body weight, at least for some people. The results of studies to date are patchy, and seem to show eating soy helps certain

---

1   It is important to note that highly processed forms of soy, such as oil, do not necessarily convey the same benefits as the whole bean.
2   Messina, M. (2016). Soy and Health Update: Evaluation of the Clinical and Epidemiologic Literature. *Nutrients*, 8(12), 754.

subgroups, not everyone. So for instance, it has been shown that soy helps weight loss in subjects who started out obese rather than people of normal weight. In the same way, soy does not generally reduce girth, but may do in people over 50.

The anti-inflammatory properties of isoflavones have been addressed in animals, cell cultures and clinical trials. The mechanisms are not entirely clear, but one of the main ones seems to be that isoflavones inhibit the genes that macrophages read to make cytokines. In addition to in vitro evidence, isoflavones suppress pro-inflammatory cytokines and chemokines during inflammatory reactions in diverse animal models and humans. Both population studies and laboratory experiments show isoflavones, particularly one called genistein, are beneficial for patients with cardiovascular diseases and cancer.

Genistein in high doses changes DNA methylation in eight-week-old mice.[3] It activates genes that suppress prostate cancer. It has similar effects on genes that regulate cancers of the breast and kidney. Early evidence suggests these beneficial changes can be passed from parents to offspring.

Cancer cells have to divide for a tumour to grow, and cancer researchers are forever looking for ways to stop them doing so. In controlled laboratory conditions, genistein inhibits division in various lines of cancer cells, including breast, prostate, hepatic, pancreatic, cervical and kidney. It even has the interesting characteristic of stopping new blood vessels forming. Tumours make their own blood vessels, as they need nutrients to grow, and strangling their supply lines is a useful treatment tactic. Genistein and another isoflavone called daidzein, in laboratory conditions, kill off developing new blood vessels as effectively as the notorious drug thalidomide, which has outstanding

---

3   Guerrero-Bosagna, C.M., & Skinner, M.K. (2012). Environmental Epigenetics and Phytoestrogen/Phytochemical Exposures. *The Journal of Steroid Biochemistry and Molecular Biology*, 139.

ability in this respect.[4] These observations are somewhat artificial, as they cannot be directly translated to the metabolism of people who eat soy as a whole food, but they are thought-provoking, and a relevant parallel to the cancer protection shown in population studies. Like other legumes, whole soy beans can be used as the protein in stew or salad. They are poisonous raw, however, and must be simmered for several hours. The immature green beans are called edamame, and are often eaten steamed in their pods. Soy sauce and miso have a lot of salt, and soy oil is high in omega-6 fatty acids.[5] All should be used sparingly. Tofu, which is fermented bean curd, like milk-free cheese, is another popular and versatile option. It is often cut into cubes and used like meat.

References

Akhlaghi, M., Zare, M., & Nouripour, F. (2017). Effect of Soy and Soy Isoflavones on Obesity-Related Anthropometric Measures: A Systematic Review and Meta-analysis of Randomized Controlled Clinical Trials. *Advances in Nutrition,* 8(5), 705-717.

Applegate, C.C., Rowles, J.L., Ranard, K.M., Jeon, S., & Erdman, J.W. (2018) Soy Consumption and the Risk of Prostate Cancer: An Updated Systematic Review and Meta-Analysis. *Nutrients,* 10(1),

Barnes, S. (2010). The Biochemistry, Chemistry and Physiology of the Isoflavones in Soybeans and their Food Products. *Lymphatic Research and Biology,* 8(1), 89-98.

Cederroth, C., & Nef, S. (2009). Soy, phytoestrogens and metabolism: A review. *Molecular and Cellular Endocrinology,* 304(1), 30-42.

Guerrero-Bosagna, C.M., & Skinner, M.K. (2012). Environmental Epigenetics and Phytoestrogen/Phytochemical Exposures. *The Journal of Steroid Biochemistry and Molecular Biology,* 139.

Hoffman, J.R., & Falvo, M.J. (2004). Protein - Which is Best? *Journal of Sports Science and Medicine,* 3(3), 118-30.

Kucuk, O. (2017). Soy foods, isoflavones, and breast cancer. *Cancer,* 123(11), 1901-1903.

Lecomte, S., Demay, F., Ferrière, F., & Pakdel, F. (2017). Phytochemicals Targeting Estrogen Receptors: Beneficial Rather Than Adverse Effects? *International Journal of Molecular Sciences,* 18(7).

---

4 Virk-Baker, M.K., Nagy, T.R., & Barnes, S. (2010). Role of phytoestrogens in cancer therapy. *Planta medica,* 76(11), 1132-1142.
5 See Omega-3 or not omega-3, that is the question.

Messina, M. (2016). Soy and Health Update: Evaluation of the Clinical and Epidemiologic Literature. *Nutrients*, 8(12), 754.

Munro, I., Harwood, M., Hlywka, J., Stephen, A., Doull, J., Flamm, W., & Adlercreutz, H. (2003). Soy Isoflavones: a Safety Review. *Nutrition Reviews*, 61(1), 1-33.

Ramdath, D.D., Padhi, E.M.T., Sarfaraz, S., Renwick, S., & Duncan, A.M. (2017). Beyond the Cholesterol-Lowering Effect of Soy Protein: A Review of the Effects of Dietary Soy and Its Constituents on Risk Factors for Cardiovascular Disease. *Nutrients*, 9(4).

Rizzo, G., & Baroni, L. (2018). Soy, Soy Foods and Their Role in Vegetarian Diets. *Nutrients*, 10(1), 43.

Setchell, K. (2017). The history and basic science development of soy isoflavones. *Menopause*, 24(12), 1338-1350.

Setchell, K. (1998). Phytoestrogens: the biochemistry, physiology, and implications for human health of soy isoflavones. *The American Journal of Clinical Nutrition*, 68(6), 1333S.

Varinska, L., Gal, P., Mojzisova, G., Mirossay, L., & Mojzis, J. (2015). Soy and Breast Cancer: Focus on Angiogenesis. Srivastava SK, ed. *International Journal of Molecular Sciences*, 16(5), 11728-11749.

Virk-Baker, M.K., Nagy, T.R., & Barnes, S. (2010). Role of phytoestrogens in cancer therapy. *Planta medica*, 76(11), 1132-1142.

Wang, Q., Ge, X., Tian, X., Zhang, Y., Zhang, J., & Zhang, P. (2013). Soy isoflavone: The multipurpose phytochemical (Review). *Biomedical Reports*, 1(5), 697-701.

Xiao, Y., Zhang, S., Tong, H., & Shi, S. (2018). Comprehensive evaluation of the role of soy and isoflavone supplementation in humans and animals over the past two decades. *Phytotherapy Research*, 32(3), 384-394.

Yu, J., Bi, X., Yu, B., & Chen, D. (2016). Isoflavones: Anti-Inflammatory Benefit and Possible Caveats. *Nutrients*, 8(6), 361.

31

CHINESE TRADITIONAL
Wormwood, skullcap and wolfberries

In 1954, a delegation from the British Labour party went to China. For its time, it was an innovative move and, as the Chinese leadership hoped, helped open Western eyes to what was going on there. It was followed by a piece in English medical journal *The Lancet*, which argued that the claims of traditional Chinese medicine, the world's oldest medical system, were 'worth investigation'.[1] Historians mark this paper as the start of a process which, by fits and starts – and hostage to cycles in Chinese politics, like the Cultural Revolution – has passed folk medicines that the Chinese have relied on for thousands of years through modern laboratories. Serious advances have resulted, including camptothecin for cancer, arsenic trioxide for leukaemia, and artemisinin for malaria—which won the Nobel prize for medicine in 2015. The task is huge and ongoing, but continues to identify bioactives of significance, including ones with long term anti-inflammatory import.[2]

Wormwood is the common name for shrubs from a genus called *Artemisia*. *Artemisia dracunculus* (or 'little dragon' from the shape of

---

1 James, D.W. (1955). Chinese medicine. *Lancet*, 265, 1068–1069.
2 Some qualifications: None of the material in this chapter is offered to suggest that the plants discussed will, when taken in supplement form, treat established disease. Skull cap and wormwood and related preparations are unsuitable in pregnancy, and for people on the clot-preventing drug Warfarin.

its leaves) is the herb tarragon, which contains numerous polyphenol flavonoids. *Artemisia absinthium* is famous for the bitter taste in green absinthe, the bilious green botanical spirit that inspired Van Gogh and Oscar Wilde. It is also a potent free radical scavenger, at least in laboratory conditions.

Their relative is *Artemisia annua,* known as sweet wormwood, whose derivatives treat malaria via the useful property of killing infected red blood cells (the malaria parasite lives in red blood cells) and leaving healthy ones alone. These derivatives also kill viruses, intestinal worms (hence the name), and cancer cells. Sweet wormwood was turned from a folk remedy to a mainstream drug by researchers in China in the 1970s, after the call went out to treat malaria in soldiers during the Vietnam war. The artemisinin they isolated remains one of the world's most effective anti-malarials. Wormwood derivatives show great promise on the cancer ward too.

Sweet wormwood acts on multiple components of the immune system, with a synergistic suppressive effect on inflammation and autoimmune diseases. Its constituents suppress inflammation in lab rats with infections, arthritis and pancreatitis, probably by blocking NF-κB.[3] They interfere with the white blood cells called macrophages, and tip the balance of cytokine production towards anti-inflammatory ones. They inhibit pathogenic white T and B cells and their associated antibodies, and expand numbers of regulatory T cells, the net result of which is anti-inflammatory. Artemisinin family molecules have even been reported effective in mouse models of asthma.[4]

Most of the research literature describes the drug side of things, but behind the power of purified molecules lies the original complex

---

3 Shakir, L., Hussain, M., Javeed, A., Ashraf, M., & Riaz, A. (2011). Artemisinins and immune system. *European Journal of Pharmacology,* 668(1), 6-14.
4 Hou, L., & Huang, H. (2016). Immune Suppressive Properties of Artemisinin Family Drugs. *Pharmacology & Therapeutics,* 166, 123-127.

plant tissue. All parts of sweet wormwood – root, leaf and flower – contain high levels of antioxidant polyphenols. They can be consumed as capsules or oil, but the least processed way is to drink an infusion as tea. Be warned, it is bitter.

Another Chinese herbal getting particular attention is *Scutellariae baicalensis Georgi*, a member of the *Scutellaria* genus, which are part of the mint family, and known as skullcaps, from the helmet shape of their flowers. Skullcaps grow all over the world, but *Scutellariae baicalensis Georgi*, better known as Baikal skullcap, grows between Siberia and Eastern Asia. Its woody carrot-shaped root is a granddaddy herb of traditional Chinese medicine.

The dried root[5] has six active flavonoid polyphenols that go by poetic names like wogonin and baicalein. They all scavenge free radicals and inhibit nitric oxide. They stop blood vessels turning leaky when inflammatory stimuli tell them to. Baicalein binds to cytokines to stop them working. Like turmeric, it makes fruit flies live longer.[6] Wogonin blocks an enzyme called cyclooxygenase-2, which is part of the production line for making inflammatory mediators from prostaglandins. A whole class of conventional anti-inflammatory drugs operate on the same enzyme. By this means, topical wogonin reduces skin rashes and inflammatory swelling in mice.[7]

The six key polyphenols collectively seem to protect brain tissue from oxidative stress and age-related neurodegeneration. Animals fed Baikal skullcap beforehand live longer when their carotid arteries, the main conduit to the brain, are tied off.[8] Baicalein breaks down brain

---

5   Sometimes referred to in the literature as *Scutellariae radix*. Radix means root.
6   Gao, L., Duan, D., Zhang, J., Zhou, Y., Qin, X., & Du, G. (2016). A Bioinformatic Approach for the Discovery of Antiaging Effects of Baicalein from Scutellaria baicalensis Georgi. *Rejuvenation Research*, 414-422.
7   Park, B., Heo, M., Park, H., & Kim, H. (2001). Inhibition of TPA-induced cyclooxygenase-2 expression and skin inflammation in mice by wogonin, a plant flavone from Scutellaria radix. *European Journal of Pharmacology*, 425(2), 153-157.
8   Zhang, Y., et al. (2006). Protective effect of flavonoids from Scutellaria baicalensis Georgi on cerebral ischemia injury. *Journal of Ethnopharmacology*, 108(3), 355-360.

amyloid deposits, the lesion behind Alzheimer's dementia. Another skullcap flavone, oroxylin A, greatly improved cognitive functions in animal models of ageing brains, and wogonin even seems to stimulate brain regeneration.[9]

A tactic of modern medicine is to give drugs that burst open the blood clots behind strokes and heart attacks. If done soon enough, this can rescue brain and heart tissue before it dies. Unfortunately, blood floods back in when the clot is busted, and a backlash of oxidative stress and inflammation can result. When this is done experimentally, both brains and hearts show less injury in animals pre-dosed with skullcap.[10]

Skullcap polyphenols show promise with cancer, particularly wogonin. They kill several different types of leukaemia cells in the laboratory, and leave normal ones alone. Work is under way to investigate clues it may have some role against solid cancers, including major killers like bowel and breast.[11]

Another ancient therapeutic, which was recorded as a remedy well over a thousand years ago, is *Lycium barbarum* or wolfberry, fruit of the boxthorn bush. Also known as the Goji berry, it is sold as a wrinkled orange raisin,[12] and can be eaten much the same way: sprinkled on cereal, blended in a smoothie or stuffed into roast turkey. It also comes as juice or tea.

One study of 50 people aged 55 to 72 years randomly fed subjects a standardised Goji preparation or placebo, so the subjects (and the professionals monitoring them) did not know who was getting the real

9 Gasiorowski, K., et al. (2011). Flavones from root of Scutellaria baicalensis Georgi: drugs of the future in neurode-generation? *CNS & Neurological Disorders-Drug Targets (Formerly Current Drug Targets-CNS & Neurological Disorders)*, 10(2), 184-191.

10 Chan, E., et al. (2011). Extract of Scutellaria baicalensis Georgi root exerts protection against myocardial is-chemia-reperfusion injury in rats. *The American Journal of Chinese Medicine*, 39(04), 693-704.

11 Wu, X., Zhang, H., Salmani, J., Fu, R., & Chen, B. (2016). Advances of wogonin, an extract from Scutellaria baicalensis , for the treatment of multiple tumors. *OncoTargets and Therapy*, 9, 2935-2943.

12 Sometimes the cheaper brands are stabilised with sulphites, which some people can be allergic to. (Buy better quality, if so).

thing. After 30 days, when the codes were broken, and the statistics were run, people who got the real thing had significant improvement in their blood-borne antioxidant enzymes.[13] Other human studies associate Goji berries with improved well-being and immune function. They also inhibit tumours in mice and protect liver and brain from induced toxic insults. They ameliorate the symptoms of mice with Alzheimer's disease. I emphasise that the claims of laboratory studies are interesting but not proof, and that anyone with an established condition like cancer needs treatment, not supplements. However, the potent anti-inflammatory properties of some of the items in the traditional Chinese pharmacopoeia imply they can make a useful contribution to an age-resisting lifestyle.

References

Aglarova, A., Zilfikarov, I., & Severtseva, O. (2008). Biological characteristics and useful properties of tarragon (Artemisia dracunculus L.) *Pharmaceutical Chemistry Journal*, 42(2), 81-86.

Alesaeidi, S., & Miraj, S. (2016). A Systematic Review of Anti-malarial Properties, Immunosuppressive Properties, Anti-inflammatory Properties, and Anti-cancer Properties of Artemisia Annua. *Electronic Physician*, 8(10), 3150-3155.

Amagase, H., Sun, B., & Borek, C. (2009). Lycium barbarum (goji) juice improves in vivo antioxidant biomarkers in serum of healthy adults. *Nutrition Research*, 29: 19-25.

Canadanovic-Brunet, J., Djilas, S., Cetkovic, G., & Tumbas, V. (2005). Free-radical scavenging activity of wormwood (Artemisia absinthium L) extracts. *Journal of the Science of Food and Agriculture*, 85(2), 265-272.

Cao, Y., et al. (2011). Baicalin attenuates global cerebral ischemia/reperfusion injury in gerbils via anti-oxidative and anti-apoptotic pathways. *Brain Research Bulletin*, 85(6)396-402.

Chan, E., et al. (2011). Extract of Scutellaria baicalensis Georgi root exerts protection against myocardial ischemia-reperfusion injury in rats. *The American Journal of Chinese Medicine*, 39(04), 693-704.

Cheng, J., Zhou, Z.W., Sheng, H.P., et al. (2014). An evidence-based update on the pharmacological activities and possible molecular targets of Lycium barbarum polysaccharides. *Drug Design, Development and Therapy*, 9, 33-78.

---

13   Amagase, H., Sun, B., & Borek, C. (2009). Lycium barbarum (goji) juice improves in vivo antioxidant biomarkers in serum of healthy adults. *Nutrition Research*, 29: 19-25.

Chi, Y-S., et al. (2003). Effects of wogonin, a plant flavone from Scutellaria radix, on skin inflammation: in vivo regulation of inflammation-associated gene expression. *Biochemical Pharmacology*, 66(7), 1271-1278.

Efferth, T. (2017). From ancient herb to modern drug: Artemisia annua and artemisinin for cancer therapy. *Seminars in Cancer Biology*, 46, 65-83.

Gao, Y., Wei, Y., Wang, Y., Gao, F., & Chen, Z. (2018). Lycium Barbarum: A Traditional Chinese Herb and A Promising Anti-Aging Agent. *Aging and Disease*, 8(6), 778-791.

Gao, Z., et al. (1999). Free radical scavenging and antioxidant activities of flavonoids extracted from the radix of Scutellaria baicalensis Georgi. *Biochimica et Biophysica Acta (BBA)-General Subjects* 1472(3), 643-650.

Gasiorowski, K., et al. (2011). Flavones from root of Scutellaria baicalensis Georgi: drugs of the future in neurodegeneration? *CNS & Neurological Disorders-Drug Targets (Formerly Current Drug Targets-CNS & Neurological Disorders)*, 10(2), 184-191.

Huang, W-H., Lee, A-R., & Yang, C-H. (2006). Antioxidative and anti-inflammatory activities of polyhydroxyflavonoids of Scutellaria baicalensis GEORGI. *Bioscience, Biotechnology, and Biochemistry*, 70(10), 2371-2380.

Hou, L., & Huang, H. (2016). Immune Suppressive Properties of Artemisinin Family Drugs. *Pharmacology & Therapeutics*, 166, 123-127.

James, D.W. (1955). Chinese medicine. *Lancet*, 265, 1068–1069.

Kayani, W.K., Kiani, B.H., Dilshad, E., & Mirza, B. (2018). Biotechnological approaches for artemisinin production in Artemisia. *World Journal of Microbiology & Biotechnology*, 34(4), 54.

Kubo, M., et al. (1984). Studies on Scutellariae radix. VII. Anti-arthritic and anti-inflammatory actions of methanolic extract and flavonoid components from Scutellariae radix. *Chemical and Pharmaceutical Bulletin*, 32(7), 2724-2729.

Li, B-Q., et al. (2000). The flavonoid baicalin exhibits anti-inflammatory activity by binding to chemokines. *Immunopharmacology*, 49(3), 295-306.

Li-Weber, M. (2009). New therapeutic aspects of flavones: The anticancer properties of Scutellaria and its main active constituents Wogonin, Baicalein and Baicalin. *Cancer Treatment Reviews*, 35(1), 57-68.

Pang, K., & Zhong, Z. (2011). Pharmacological effects and pharmacokinetics properties of Radix Scutellariae and its bioactive flavones. *Biopharmaceutics and Drug Disposition*, 32(8), 427-445.

Park, B., Heo, M., Park, H., & Kim, H. (2001). Inhibition of TPA-induced cyclooxygenase-2 expression and Skin inflammation in mice by wogonin, a plant flavone from Scutellaria radix. *European Journal of Pharmacology*, 425(2), 153-157.

Polier, G., et al. (2011). Wogonin and related natural flavones are inhibitors of CDK9 that induce apoptosis in cancer cells by transcriptional suppression of Mcl-1. *Cell Death & Disease*, 2(7), e182.

Reichek, N., & Parcham-Azad, K. (2010). Reperfusion Injury. *Journal of the American College of Cardiology*, 55(12), 1206-1208.

Shakir, L., Hussain, M., Javeed, A., Ashraf, M., & Riaz, A. (2011). Artemisinins and immune system. *European Journal of Pharmacology*, 668(1), 6-14.

Shi, C., Li, H., Yang, Y., & Hou, L. (2015). Anti-Inflammatory and Immunoregulatory Functions of Artemisinin and Its Derivatives. *Mediators of Inflammation*.

Song, Y., Desta, K., Kim, G., Lee, S., Lee, W., Kim, Y., Jin, J., Abd El-Aty, A., Shin, H., Shim, J., & Shin, S. (2016). Polyphenolic profile and antioxidant effects of various parts of Artemisia annua L. *Biomedical Chromatography*, 30(4), 588-595.

Van Noorden, R. (2010). Demand for malaria drug soars. *Nature*, 466(7307), 672-673.

Wright, P. (2010). Passport to Peking: A very British mission to Mao's China. Oxford: Oxford University Press.

Wu, X., Zhang, H., Salmani, J., Fu, R., & Chen, B. (2016). Advances of wogonin, an extract from Scutellaria baicalensis, for the treatment of multiple tumors. *OncoTargets and Therapy*, 9, 2935-2943.

Xu, Q., Bauer, R., Hendry, B.M., et al. (2013). The quest for modernisation of traditional Chinese medicine. *BMC Complementary and Alternative Medicine*, 13,132.

Zhang, Y., et al. (2006). Protective effect of flavonoids from Scutellaria baicalensis Georgi on cerebral ischemia injury. *Journal of Ethnopharmacology*, 108(3), 355-360.

32

ELIXIR OF THE AZTECS
The serious side of chocolate

Chocolate is bad for health and weight, and should only be eaten as a treat; except it isn't, and should be eaten for good health and long life. Or at least it should be if the original, bitter, lightly processed drink of the Aztec Indians could be recreated. Cacao beans have as many antioxidants as fruit and vegetables, but modern chocolate in bars and coloured boxes does not. Modern chocolate is a refined and roasted remnant of cacao beans, enhanced with sugar, milk powder and oil. But, unfortunately, that is how we like it.

When chocolate first came to Europe in the sixteenth century, commercial minds soon saw the potential of removing the bitterness and making it palatable. Pharmacies and food shops experimented with cooking and spices which enthused the public and opened their purses; the process has continued since. Chocolate has considerable potential to deliver longevity, but it only moves off shop shelves as a mouthful of unctuous sweetness, or a coating for nuts and soft centres. A better example of nature's gift ruined by the free market, there is none.

The vital part of chocolate is the cocoa solids, which are principally bitter polyphenols, like the ones in wine and tea. Numerous studies show that cocoa solids promote good health and long life.[1] Cocoa solids

1 Ellam, S., & Williamson, G. (2013). Cocoa and Human Health. *Annual Review of Nutrition*, 33, 105-128.

are the difference between light and dark chocolate, and the reason dark chocolate is the healthiest. Chocolate makers know you know that and make liberal and unregulated use of the word 'dark' on their labels. Chocolate starts with beans from cacao trees[2] which grow, 30 or 40 at a time, inside fibrous pods shaped like rugby balls. The beans are too bitter to eat, so after harvest they are piled underneath the trees for a few days to get warm. In this first step, called fermentation, enzymes from bacteria and yeast smooth out the astringency, which means they destroy some of the polyphenols. Further steps destroy more. Fermented beans are dried to preserve them, in ovens or the open air, then roasted at high temperatures. The fibrous shells are removed with violent shaking, which leaves fragments called nibs, which are the edible bit. What happens after the nibs appear is complex, but, in simple terms, ground-up nibs, with various amounts of sugar, fat and milk powder ('milk chocolate') become chocolate bars. About half the volume of nibs is fat, called cocoa butter, which has the useful quality – ideal for a food fat – of turning from solid to liquid at mouth temperature. The rest is cocoa solids, including the all-important polyphenols.

Chocolate polyphenols are from a polyphenol class called flavonoids, particularly one called epicatechin, and cocoa is one of the very richest sources of them. Among other things, they appear to preserve mitochondria, the cell furnaces whose failure is central to the inflammage, and blood vessel linings (atherosclerosis starts when ruptured linings admit cholesterol; see Keeping the lines open). Various lines of research show chocolate polyphenols block numerous elements of the immune system, such as cytokines and NF-κB.

---

2   The literature often refers to cocoa beans and cocoa trees, but it appears best practice is to use cacao – after the tree *Theobroma cacao* – for beans and trees, and cocoa for the fat-free powder that appears later in the manufacturing process. https://en.oxforddictionaries.com/definition/cocoa. See also the definitions in Ellam, S., & Williamson, G. (2013). Cocoa and human health. *Annual Review of Nutrition*, 33, 105–128.

Unfortunately, they are killed off by fermentation, roasting and all the other steps that make chocolate as we know it. Flavonoids are particularly destroyed by 'dutching', a common step in making commercial grade chocolate, which uses alkalis to neutralise acid left over from fermentation.

A dramatic example of chocolate's properties is provided by the Kuna Indians who live on the San Blas islands, off the coast of Panama, and who regularly drink unprocessed chocolate from their own trees. That means they consume far more, and better quality, than their compatriots on the mainland who get theirs from supermarkets. In 2007, a study of death certificates from 2000 to 2004 was undertaken to probe the causes of mortality in the region. It found the Kuna, compared to the mainland people, had dramatically lower rates of heart disease, stroke, cancer and diabetes.[3] A study like this can't prove what causes the difference – a common issue with comparative studies – but the Kuna's highly individual chocolate diet seems likely to play a part.

Similar observations have been made elsewhere. There do not appear to be other subjects who drink the traditional formula, but research on modern diets shows even the commercial version, despite the degradations of processing, retains some of its power. A questionnaire evaluation of almost 5,000 people in the United States aged from their twenties to their nineties, found that people who ate less chocolate were more likely to have heart disease.[4] The same research group, in a different exercise, stuck over 2,000 people under a scanner and measured the calcium around their hearts, a known way

3   Bayard, V., Chamorro, F., Motta, J., & Hollenberg, N.K. (2007). Does Flavanol Intake Influence Mortality from Nitric Oxide-Dependent Processes? Ischemic Heart Disease, Stroke, Diabetes Mellitus, and Cancer in Panama. *International Journal of Medical Sciences*, 4(1), 53-58.
4   Djoussé L, Hopkins PN, North KE, Pankow JS, Arnett DK, Ellison RC. (2011). Chocolate Consumption is Inversely Associated with Prevalent Coronary Heart Disease: The National Heart, Lung, and Blood Institute Family Heart Study. *Clinical Nutrition (Edinburgh, Scotland)*, 30(2), 182-187.

of estimating critical fat deposits in coronary arteries (fat deposits, or atherosclerosis, become calcified over time: see <u>Keeping the lines open</u>). They found the chocolate-eaters had less of them.[5] Another study that followed several hundred elderly Dutch men over fifteen years found the chocolate-eaters had lower blood pressure, healthier hearts and longer lives.[6] A similar study in the medieval city of Porto, in Portugal, followed several hundred subjects over 65 years of age and found that, over a period of four years, cognitive decline was lower for chocolate-eaters.[7] Patients in Sweden presenting to hospital with their first heart attack had a better chance of surviving long term if they were chocolate-eaters.[8] Another study of a large group showed chocolate-eaters had lower levels of blood-borne markers of inflammation.[9]

When various studies of this type were combined, what epidemiologists call a meta-analysis, the risk of heart attacks and strokes totted up across them was lower among those who ate modest amounts of chocolate.[10]

So chocolate is not merely an indulgent treat if used judiciously, and the over-processed, sugar and fat-laden pitfalls are avoided. Flavonoids are astringent, so some accommodation with taste-enhancers is inevitable, and the challenge is finding a balance. Chocolate nibs can

5   Djoussé, L., Hopkins, P.N., Arnett, D.K., et al. (2011). Chocolate Consumption is Inversely Associated with Calcified Atherosclerotic Plaque in the Coronary Arteries: The NHLBI Family Heart Study. *Clinical Nutrition (Edinburgh, Scotland)*, 30(1), 38-43.
6   Buijsse, B., Feskens, E., Kok, F., & Kromhout, D. (2006). Cocoa Intake, Blood Pressure, and Cardiovascular Mortality. The Zutphen Elderly Study. *JAMA Internal Medicine*, 166(4), 411-417.
7   Moreira, A., Diógenes, M., de Mendonça, A., Lunet, N., & Barros, H. (2016). Chocolate Consumption is Associated with a Lower Risk of Cognitive Decline. *Journal of Alzheimer's Disease*, 53(1), 85-93.
8   Janszky, I., Mukamal, K., Ljung, R., Ahnve, S., Ahlbom, A., & Hallqvist, J. (2009). Chocolate consumption and mortality following a first acute myocardial infarction: the Stockholm Heart Epidemiology Program. *Journal of Internal Medicine*, 266(3).
9   Khan N, Khymenets O, Urpí-Sardà M, et al. (2014). Cocoa Polyphenols and Inflammatory Markers of Cardiovascular Disease. *Nutrients*, 6(2), 844-880.
10 Gianfredi, V., Salvatori, T., Nucci, D., Villarini, M., & Moretti, M. (2018). Can chocolate consumption reduce cardio-cerebrovascular risk? A systematic review and meta-analysis. *Nutrition*, 46, 103-114.

be purchased. They are half cacao bean fat, but are lightly processed, additive free, and easily folded into smoothies and nut mixes. Chocolate bars cover a range, so look at the fine print. Avoid anything 'dutched' in favour of more flavonol-friendly processes like conching.[11] Look past the word 'dark', which means not much, to the percentage of cocoa solids. Hold out for seventy per cent and above.

References
Bayard, V., Chamorro, F., Motta, J., & Hollenberg, N.K. (2007). Does Flavanol Intake Influence Mortality from Nitric Oxide-Dependent Processes? Ischemic Heart Disease, Stroke, Diabetes Mellitus, and Cancer in Panama. *International Journal of Medical Sciences*, 4(1), 53-58.

Blumberg, J., Ding, E., Dixon, R., Pasinetti, G., & Villarreal, F. (2014). The Science of Cocoa Flavanols: Bioavailability, Emerging Evidence, and Proposed Mechanisms. *Advances in Nutrition*, 5(5), 547-549.

Buijsse, B., Feskens, E., Kok, F., & Kromhout, D. (2006). Cocoa Intake, Blood Pressure, and Cardiovascular Mortality. The Zutphen Elderly Study. *JAMA Internal Medicine*, 166(4), 411-417.

De Vuyst, L. and Weckx, S. (2016), The cocoa bean fermentation process: from ecosystem analysis to starter culture development. *Journal of Applied Microbiology*, 121, 5–17.

Di Mattia, C.D., Sacchetti, G., Mastrocola, D., & Serafini, M. (2017). From Cocoa to Chocolate: The Impact of Processing on *In Vitro* Antioxidant Activity and the Effects of Chocolate on Antioxidant Markers *In Vivo*. *Frontiers in Immunology*, 8(1207).

Djoussé L, Hopkins PN, North KE, Pankow JS, Arnett DK, Ellison RC. (2011). Chocolate Consumption is Inversely Associated with Prevalent Coronary Heart Disease: The National Heart, Lung, and Blood Institute Family Heart Study. *Clinical Nutrition, (Edinburgh, Scotland)*, 30(2), 182-187.

Djoussé, L., Hopkins, P.N., Arnett, D.K., et al. (2011). Chocolate Consumption is Inversely Associated with Calcified Atherosclerotic Plaque in the Coronary Arteries: The NHLBI Family Heart Study. *Clinical Nutrition (Edinburgh, Scotland)*, 30(1), 38-43.

Ellam, S., & Williamson, G. (2013). Cocoa and Human Health. *Annual Review of Nutrition*, 33, 105-128.

Gianfredi, V., Salvatori, T., Nucci, D., Villarini, M., & Moretti, M. (2018). Can chocolate consumption reduce cardio-cerebrovascular risk? A systematic review and meta-analysis. *Nutrition*, 46, 103-114.

Higginbotham, E., & Taub, P. (2015). Cardiovascular Benefits of Dark Chocolate? *Current Treatment Options in Cardiovascular Medicine*, 17(12), 1-12.

---

11   Conching is named after a conche, or shell, and refers to a vessel in which liquid chocolate is gently heated and agitated for an extended period so that undesirable flavours evaporate and the cocoa butter is evenly mixed with the solid particles.

Hurst, W., Krake, S., Bergmeier, S., Payne, M., Miller, K., & Stuart, D. (2011). Impact of fermentation, drying, roasting and Dutch processing on flavan-3-ol stereochemistry in cacao beans and cocoa ingredients. *Chemistry Central Journal, 5*(1), 1-10.

Janszky, I., Mukamal, K., Ljung, R., Ahnve, S., Ahlbom, A., & Hallqvist, J. (2009). Chocolate consumption and mortality following a first acute myocardial infarction: the Stockholm Heart Epidemiology Program. *Journal of Internal Medicine, 266*(3),

Khan N, Khymenets O, Urpí-Sardà M, et al. (2014). Cocoa Polyphenols and Inflammatory Markers of Cardiovascular Disease. *Nutrients, 6*(2), 844-880.

McShea, A., Ramiro-Puig, E., Munro, S., Casadesus, G., Castell, M., & Smith, M. (2008). Clinical benefit and preservation of flavonols in dark chocolate manufacturing. *Nutrition Reviews, 66*(11), 630-641.

Moreira, A., Diógenes, M., de Mendonça, A., Lunet, N., & Barros, H. (2016). Chocolate Consumption is Associated with a Lower Risk of Cognitive Decline. *Journal of Alzheimer's Disease, 53*(1), 85-93.

Petyaev, I.M., & Bashmakov, Y.K. (2017). Dark Chocolate: Opportunity for an Alliance between Medical Science and the Food Industry? *Frontiers in Nutrition, 4*(43).

S Rössner (1997). Chocolate—divine food, fattening junk or nutritious supplementation? *European Journal of Clinical Nutrition,* 51, 341–345

https://en.oxforddictionaries.com/definition/cocoa.

FROM WORDS TO DEEDS
Pulling it all together

So food is not just nutrition. Protein, carbohydrates and vitamins keep you going, but the best and most wholesome food is more. The right food medicates you, and good health and long life means a daily dose of the right options. In particular, the right food medicates your immune system, and forestalls as long as possible the inflammatory imbalance that underpins life's common catastrophic diseases.

The concepts I have laid out have plenty of room in them for argument, which I hope I have adequately acknowledged. Some health authorities will turn purple at the claims in these pages, and others will quietly opine that there is no evidence to support them. Which is not true, of course. There is no conclusive evidence everyone can agree on, but the same can be said of many of the scientific world's big issues. However, there is more than enough evidence to engage thoughtful and open-minded people, and such people do not need certainty to recognise relevance. There is always a new horizon after the last one has been crossed, and since researchers have shown certain patterns of eating are healthy, finding and concentrating the elements that do the work is the next obvious step.

In the end, having the debate, and pricking the establishment, is half the fun. Nobody writes books anymore arguing that smoking is bad for you; where that debate once raged, consensus reigns and everyone has moved on. Settled ideas are useful to know, but it is new thinking that draws in the mind and quickens the pulse. The parameters of knowledge advance only when enough people are willing to look beyond orthodoxy. Being part of the journey is stimulating.

I have done my best to render the science comprehensible, but for those interested in my sources each chapter of this book, as you have seen, ends with a list of the journal papers used to write it. In addition crucial statements, like individual studies, have their own numbered reference. I have tried to keep the numbered references to a minimum, as they interrupt the text but the important ones have to be there for credibility. Anyone interested can find most of these papers on PubMed (https://www.ncbi.nlm.nih.gov/pubmed/), which is a free search engine that accesses a huge life sciences database maintained by the United States National Library of Medicine.

Ultimately, however, the central issue for most people, after reading this far, is how these insights can be implemented. The answer is personal and individual, but there are guiding principles.

The first is not to take on any lifestyle revolution that you are not going to maintain. Bean sprouts and salmon every night will pall after a while, as will turmeric and chillies in every dish, and anything else for which long-term enthusiasm can't be guaranteed. Likewise with exercise. A walk around the block every morning matters more than a gym membership that lasts three months.

At the simplest end, don't make things worse. That means do not eat highly processed food. Highly processed food satisfies your hunger without delivering the array of crucial anti-inflammatory polyphenols that lightly cooked plants do. It is also a major vector for white flour and refined sugar which, as you have read, stirs up inflammation and puts fat in the wrong places.

Remember that dangerous fat deposits are not substantial. Do not take comfort from a normal body weight if you are not eating well (and don't despair if your weight remains stubbornly high if you are). The next step is to add some new, bioactive-rich food to your regular diet: a tin of sardines once a week can be accommodated by most people if they put their minds to it, as can a square of dark chocolate a day, and a glass of pomegranate juice. Likewise a regular place can be found for rolled oat porridge, tofu, and plenty of non-salt seasoning. Any number of similar simple measures based on the preceding chapters will improve your inflammatory balance without throwing your domestic routine into disarray.

Ultimately, however, the functional food philosophy implies a place for complex, food-like supplements. A carefully defined place, but a viable one nonetheless. Grape seeds and olive leaves and various other useful and powerful options are difficult to eat regularly any other way. My own company, LifeGuard Health®, makes a supplement of five major bioactives: turmeric (with piperine), olive leaf extract, grape seed and skin extract, boswellia and skull cap. The website www.lifeguard. health provides ordering details, as well as further information about the ingredients, other outlets that sell it, and regular posts about the anti-inflammatory lifestyle. The five ingredients are the ones, it seems to me, that are foremost among the options that can't be efficiently accessed via whole food. They are therefore just what you need for that extra anti-inflammatory boost if you are already eating sensibly.

Good health and long life to you.

GLOSSARY

Angiogenesis. The process of growing new blood vessels. Found in both healing tissue and cancers.

Anthocyanin. A group of polyphenol antioxidants that give plants like blueberries and pomegranate their blue and red colours.

Antioxidant. A substance that prevents oxidation. In respect of health, antioxidants remove oxidising free radicals. They are common in coloured plants, and a major reason diets that emphasise lightly processed plants are so healthy.

Atherosclerosis. A deposit of cholesterol, with associated scar tissue, in the wall of an artery. The major cause of heart attacks and strokes.

Bioactive. Food or a food derivative with biological properties beyond nutrition. A synonym for functional food.

Bioavailability. A measure of how much of something which has been eaten gets through the gut wall and past liver metabolism to enter the general circulation.

Blood-brain barrier. The barrier made by joins between the cells lining blood vessels in the brain. These joins are tighter than in other organs, and restrict which blood-borne molecules can squeeze through.

Carcinogen. A substance that causes or contributes to cancer. Tobacco, for instance.

Claudication. A pain in leg muscles caused by oxygen deficit due to exercising with partially obstructed arteries.

Cytokines. The small molecules which cells use to send messages to each other and which coordinate the process of inflammation.

Epigenetics. The process of effecting genetic-based changes by manipulating the way genes are read without altering the sequence of DNA. Comparable to choosing the pages of a book without changing the book itself.

Foam cells. White blood cells in the wall of an artery that have ingested cholesterol molecules.

Free radicals. Unstable molecules with unpaired electrons. In respect of health, they are a by-product of burning food for energy, and other lifestyle choices. They are a major cause of age-related ill health if not removed. Antioxidants neutralise them.

Functional food. A food or a food derivative with biological properties beyond nutrition. A synonym for bioactive.

Gene reader. The cellular machinery that turns the information coded in genes, or DNA sequences, into proteins.

Histones. Protein spools that DNA winds around which control how it is read. Manipulating histones is a technique of epigenetics.

Hormesis. The principle that something usually toxic like radiation or a chemical can be beneficial in a small dose.

Immune system. The diffuse collection of organs (like spleen and tonsils), blood cells and specialised proteins (like antibodies) that resists infections and repairs physical insults.

Inflammation. A set response of the immune system that mobilises white blood cells and specialised proteins to the site of an infection or physical insult.

Methylation. The process of inserting a molecule called a methyl group into a sequence of DNA so it can't be read. A technique of epigenetics.

Mitochondria. Organelles inside cells where food molecules react with oxygen to release energy.

Neurotransmitter. A chemical which nerve cells transmit between them to create or damp down impulses. A common target for psychoactive medications.

Nuclear factor kappa B (NF-κB). A protein that controls how 400 or so genes that code for proteins of inflammation are read. It is a key bottleneck in the control process and a common point of attack for natural anti-inflammatories.

Nutraceutical. A nutrition-cum-pharmaceutical, or the active fraction of functional food in concentrated form.

Oncogene. A gene that causes or contributes to cancer.

Oxygen species. Highly reactive molecules based on the oxygen atom. Includes oxygen based free radicals.

Phagocytosis. The process of a specialised white blood cell called a phagocyte wrapping itself around a foreign body or bacteria to remove it.

Phenol. A molecule based on a ring of six carbon atoms. A common building block of plant-based nutraceuticals.

Phytochemicals. Any chemical from a plant but, in practice, the term is used to refer to those with health-giving properties.

Reactive species. The collective term for different types of free radicals and other highly reactive molecules.

Senescence. This term, when applied to a cell, means the state in which a cell stops dividing without dying. When applied to an organism it means a state of functional decline.

Sirtuins. A group of seven proteins with a key role in regulating cell metabolism, particularly in periods of stress, like calorie restriction. Certain nutraceuticals like turmeric and grape seeds are postulated to deliver some of their benefit by stimulating sirtuins. A major area of longevity research is trying to find a drug which could do the same.

Telomere. The sequence at the end of a DNA molecule which protects it like the wax caps on a shoelace. Telomeres get shorter with repeated DNA replication, and telomere failure is a major factor in senescence.

ABOUT THE AUTHOR

Roderick Mulgan has been a doctor for a quarter century and is a Fellow of the Royal New Zealand College of General Practitioners. Over the last decade he has developed a multi-doctor practice that services aged-care facilities. His aged-care work has led to an interest in the effect of lifestyle choices on well-being and in particular – unusual among mainstream doctors – the evidence that novel foods and supplements promote long-term health.

With barrister Stephen Iorns he has founded LifeGuard Health®, which markets LifeGuard Essentials®, a supplement that delivers several of the nutraceuticals outlined in this book. Stephen has both professional and personal interests in health and nutrition. Dr Mulgan is also a practising barrister, and met Stephen at Victoria University School of Law. They have worked together as barristers since 2012.

Dr Mulgan lives in Auckland, and is married with two adult daughters. For further details of LifeGuard® and its products see www.lifeguard.health.

Printed in May 2019
by Rotomail Italia S.p.A., Vignate (MI) - Italy